THE PREPPERS SURVIVAL GUIDE

A Practical Manual for Preparedness, Stockpiling and Thriving in Crisis Situations

Bernard Cage Hillary

Table of Contents

INTRODUCTION

Preparedness in Modern World

Preparedness is about being ready for unexpected situations that might affect our safety, health, or even our everyday lives. In the modern world, things like natural disasters, power outages, economic crises, and even personal emergencies can happen when we least expect it. Having a plan and knowing what to do can make a big difference in how we respond and recover.

One reason why being prepared is important is because emergencies can come in many forms, and often, they happen quickly. Think of natural events like earthquakes, floods, or wildfires. These can cause damage, cut off access to clean water, food, or electricity, and leave people without safe places to stay. Being prepared can mean having supplies on hand, like food and water, but it also means knowing how to use resources wisely so we're able to take care of ourselves and our families.

Another big part of preparedness is knowing what to expect. When we're aware of the possible risks around us, we're better equipped to handle them. For instance, if we live in a place that experiences severe weather, we can plan to have a secure area to stay during storms. Or if there's a chance of a power outage, having backup lights, extra batteries, and ways to stay warm can make a difference. Even knowing simple first-aid skills can help us care for others and ourselves if medical help isn't available right away.

Preparedness isn't just about having physical supplies. It's also about learning skills that help us feel more confident and independent. For example, knowing how to start a fire safely, build a temporary shelter, or find clean water are valuable skills that help us in difficult situations. By practicing these skills before we actually need them, we're able to stay calm and act wisely when emergencies happen. These skills don't just make us feel safer; they remind us that we're capable of taking care of ourselves even when things are uncertain.

Planning for the unexpected also builds something called "resilience," which is the ability to recover or "bounce back" after facing challenges. Resilience means that we don't get overwhelmed when things go wrong. Instead, we find solutions and keep moving forward. This kind of strength doesn't just help in emergencies; it's useful for everyday life too, as it helps us handle changes and challenges with a clear mind.

This book is meant to guide you through everything you need to know about being prepared. It covers topics like gathering essential supplies, learning survival skills, securing your home, and much more. Each chapter will take you step-by-step through important topics so you can learn how to prepare in ways that make sense for you and your family. The goal is not just to teach you how to survive in emergencies but to help you build confidence and understanding about preparedness.

When we take time to prepare, we're also helping others in our community because we're more likely to be calm, informed, and able to share what we know. Preparedness is about working together, and with the skills and plans you'll learn, you'll be ready to face challenges with knowledge, care, and strength. Whether we're facing a big storm, a power outage, or a minor accident, being prepared means we're ready to handle it with confidence and resilience.

CHAPTER 1

Understanding Preparedness

Key Threats and Risks Every Prepper Must Know

Preparedness starts with understanding the types of emergencies that can happen, and why it's important to be ready for them. These threats, whether they're large events like natural disasters or smaller personal challenges, can affect people's lives in many ways. Knowing about these threats helps us think ahead, plan, and stay safe if they do happen.

One major category of threat is natural disasters, which include events like earthquakes, hurricanes, tornadoes, floods, and wildfires. These events are powerful, can cause a lot of damage, and sometimes happen with very little warning. For example, hurricanes bring strong winds and heavy rain, which can lead to flooding, destruction of homes, and loss of power. In places where hurricanes are common, like parts of the southeastern United States, people may have a plan for what to do if one is approaching. They might have emergency kits ready and know where to find shelter. Another example is earthquakes, which can shake the ground so strongly that buildings, bridges, and roads are damaged. In places like California, where earthquakes are more frequent, people practice drills to learn how to "drop, cover, and hold on" to stay safe.

Floods are another common natural disaster. They happen when there's too much rain, or when rivers overflow. Floods can sweep away cars, damage buildings, and make it hard for people to get clean drinking water. In recent years, some areas have seen more flooding due to climate changes, which brings more intense storms and rainfall. For this reason, learning how to prepare for floods and knowing if you live in a flood-prone area is essential for preppers.

Wildfires, which are uncontrolled fires in forests or grasslands, are also becoming more common, especially in dry, hot regions. Wildfires can spread quickly, destroying homes, forcing people to evacuate, and filling the air with smoke that can be harmful to breathe. Places like California, Australia, and parts of Europe have all faced major wildfires in recent years. For people who live near forests or large fields, having a plan to evacuate and protect their homes from fire is very important.

Aside from natural disasters, another big threat that preppers consider is economic collapse. This happens when a country's economy goes through a major downturn, and people start losing their jobs, prices go up, and things become difficult to afford. In extreme cases, people might find it hard to buy food, medicine, or other essential items. One example of economic collapse happened in the

Great Depression in the 1930s when millions of people lost their jobs, and many families had to live with very little money. More recently, the economic recession of 2008 affected many countries, and some people lost their homes or struggled financially. Preparing for economic problems might include saving money, learning how to grow food, or even trading goods with neighbors to get the things they need.

Pandemics, like the COVID-19 pandemic, are another major threat. A pandemic occurs when a new disease spreads quickly across the world, affecting many people. In 2020, COVID-19 affected millions of people, leading to lockdowns, business closures, and changes in daily life. Schools and workplaces had to adjust to new ways of operating, and many people stayed home to protect their health. This event reminded people of the importance of having health supplies, like masks and hand sanitizers, and learning how to take care of health needs in an emergency. Some families also prepared by keeping extra food, medicine, and other essentials at home, knowing they might need to stay indoors for a long time.

Societal unrest is another risk that preppers think about. This can happen during times of political tension, protests, or other disruptions that lead to unsafe conditions in cities or communities. For instance, during times of protest or riots, there can be damage to property, roadblocks, and disturbances in regular services like public transportation or deliveries. Societal unrest can be unpredictable, making it important for people to stay informed and have a plan for how to keep safe, especially if they live in large cities where these events might be more likely.

Another risk that has gained attention is cyber threats. These are risks that come from people using computers to harm others, like hacking into systems, spreading false information, or stealing personal data. Cyber threats can affect things like bank accounts, electricity grids, and other important services. For example, in recent years, some cyber-attacks have targeted hospitals, banks, and even governments, causing major disruptions. While people might not always know how to prevent cyber threats themselves, they can learn ways to protect their personal information, like using strong passwords and not sharing private details online.

Food and water shortages are also concerns for preppers, especially if natural disasters or other major events interrupt the usual supply chains that bring food to stores. In times of shortage, the prices of basic items like milk, bread, and vegetables can rise, or these items might be hard to find at all. Having a stockpile of non-perishable foods, like rice, canned beans, and dried fruits, can be helpful during times when stores might not be fully stocked. Some preppers also learn to grow their own food or store water in case there's a disruption in the supply.

Power outages can be a serious problem, especially if they last for days or even weeks. Power outages might happen because of storms, accidents, or even issues with the energy grid. When the power goes out, people might lose access to heat, air conditioning, lights, or even ways to cook food. In 2021, parts of Texas experienced a winter storm that left many people without power in freezing temperatures. Events like this show the importance of being prepared with backup power sources, like generators, batteries, or alternative ways to stay warm.

Understanding these threats helps us see the value in being prepared. Each of these situations has its own challenges, and by thinking ahead, we can take steps to protect ourselves and our loved ones. Preparedness means more than just having supplies on hand; it's about learning skills, knowing how to react, and feeling confident in our ability to handle unexpected situations. For families, discussing these potential risks can help everyone understand what to do and where to go if an emergency happens.

In a world where different types of emergencies can happen, being aware and prepared is one of the best ways to stay safe and resilient. Whether it's knowing how to handle a power outage, understanding how to find clean water, or having supplies ready for a storm, preparation gives us peace of mind and the tools we need to handle whatever comes our way. Being a prepper is not about expecting the worst, but about being ready to respond wisely and safely when challenges arise.

Self-Assessment: Evaluating Your Current Preparedness Level

Assessing our preparedness level is a great way to understand how ready we are for different types of emergencies. Taking the time to go through each area of preparedness; such as food, health, home security, communication, and finances helps us identify any gaps in our plan and know where we might need to improve. This self-assessment is like a checklist that covers essential areas of readiness, helping us feel more confident in our ability to handle unexpected situations.

The first area to evaluate is food storage. In emergencies, access to stores may be limited, so having a supply of food on hand can make a big difference. Start by looking at what types of food you have stored. Do you have non-perishable items, like canned goods, rice, beans, and pasta? These types of foods can last for a long time and don't need to be kept cold. Aim to have enough food stored to last at least two weeks, if not longer. Check for variety, too, so you have a balanced mix of proteins, carbohydrates, and healthy fats. It's also important to think about cooking; if there's a power outage, will you have a way to heat food or boil water? Simple tools like a camping stove or even a fire-safe pot can come in handy for emergencies. Regularly rotating your food supply by eating and replacing items ensures they don't go bad and stay fresh.

Next, evaluate health and medical readiness. Emergencies can make it harder to reach a doctor or get medicine, so it's smart to be prepared for basic health needs. Do you have a first-aid kit that's fully stocked? Basic items to include are bandages, antiseptic wipes, pain relievers, and any prescription medications needed by family members. It's also useful to have some cold medicines, allergy pills, and other basic treatments on hand. If anyone in the family has specific health conditions, consider extra supplies they might need. Knowing basic first-aid skills, like how to clean a wound or treat a minor injury, can be very helpful. Some families also keep a list of nearby medical facilities or contacts for healthcare providers in case they need extra support.

Home security is another key area to check. Keeping our homes safe during an emergency might mean protecting it against break-ins or making sure it can withstand bad weather. Start by assessing how secure your doors and windows are. Do they have strong locks? Are there any weak points, like doors or windows that don't close well? If you live in an area prone to severe weather, think about whether your home would hold up in a storm. Simple fixes, like installing sturdy locks or having storm shutters, can add extra safety. Another layer of security could include alarm systems or cameras, which can help keep track of what's happening around your property. In emergency situations, knowing how to secure your home can give you peace of mind.

Communication is an often-overlooked part of preparedness but is incredibly important. If phone lines or the internet go down, how will you stay in touch with loved ones or get important information? It's a good idea to have a few communication options, like a portable radio to hear news updates, especially if there's no power. Two-way radios can also help family members communicate if they're separated. Make sure everyone knows who to contact and has important phone numbers written down in case mobile phones don't work. Some families create a contact plan, agreeing on a central person to check in with if they can't reach each other directly. Practicing these communication methods helps ensure they work when needed.

Financial readiness means being able to manage resources wisely in an emergency. This includes having a small amount of cash on hand since ATMs or credit cards might not work if there's a power outage. Keeping some savings in reserve for emergencies can provide a cushion if unexpected expenses come up, like needing to travel or replace essential items. It's also smart to keep important financial documents—such as insurance papers, identification, and bank records—in a secure but accessible place. Digital copies stored on a USB drive or a secure online location can provide backup if you can't reach physical copies. Budgeting for preparedness supplies and making small additions over time can help make financial readiness more manageable.

To help you identify any gaps in these areas, use a simple checklist. First, for food storage, ask yourself: Do I have enough food for two weeks? Do I have a way to cook if there's no power? Next, for health, consider: Is my first-aid kit fully stocked, and do I have extra medications? For home security, think about whether your home is secure against possible threats or weather events. For communication, make sure: Do I have a way to receive news if the internet or power goes out? Do we have a family contact plan? Lastly, for finances, ask yourself if you have some cash, savings, and access to important documents.

Regularly reviewing and updating your preparedness level is helpful because our needs and situations can change. For example, as children grow, they might need new items or different supplies. Or, if you move to a new area, you might face different types of weather or other risks. Each time you go through this self-assessment, you're reinforcing your understanding and strengthening your readiness.

Remember, preparedness is a journey, not something that happens overnight. Taking small steps in each of these areas builds up over time, giving you the confidence that you're ready for whatever comes. Knowing your strengths and identifying areas to improve helps you feel in control and gives you peace of mind. When we're prepared, we're not just protecting ourselves; we're also setting an example and helping others be more resilient in times of need. Each step you take brings you closer to being fully prepared, and with regular practice, you'll have the skills and knowledge needed to face challenges with confidence and calmness.

Developing the Right Mindset for Survival

Developing the right mindset for survival is about preparing our minds and emotions to handle tough situations calmly and confidently. While having supplies and skills is essential, our mindset plays a big role in how we respond to emergencies. Our thoughts and emotions influence our actions, so learning to be resilient, adaptable, and calm under pressure can make all the difference. These mental qualities allow us to think clearly, make smart decisions, and stay strong when things get difficult.

One key quality for survival is resilience. Resilience is the ability to bounce back from setbacks or challenges. It doesn't mean we won't feel stressed, scared, or tired, but that we're able to recover and keep going. Building resilience begins with practicing positive thinking and not giving up when things go wrong. Even in daily life, facing small challenges without getting discouraged helps us grow stronger mentally. Reminding ourselves of times when we overcame obstacles helps us believe in our strength. This self-belief becomes important in emergencies, reminding us that we can handle difficulties and find solutions.

Adaptability is another important trait for survival. In a crisis, things rarely go as planned, so we must be willing to adjust. This doesn't mean changing everything we're doing, but being flexible enough to find new ways forward if our original plan isn't working. Adaptable people see challenges as chances to learn. Instead of focusing on problems, they look for different approaches. To practice adaptability, we can try changing routines or experimenting with new solutions to minor issues we face daily. This makes us more comfortable with change and prepares us to handle unexpected events without feeling overwhelmed.

Staying calm under pressure is a skill that helps us think clearly and avoid panicking. In stressful situations, our body's "fight or flight" response can make us feel anxious or scared. While this is natural, we can learn ways to manage these feelings. Deep breathing, for example, is a simple technique that helps slow our heartbeat and relaxes our mind. When we breathe slowly, it sends a message to our brain that we're okay, allowing us to focus. Practicing this during everyday stress helps us stay calm when bigger challenges arise. Staying calm doesn't mean ignoring the problem, but approaching it with a clear and focused mind.

Another way to develop the right mindset is to set small goals, especially during challenging moments. Instead of feeling overwhelmed by everything at once, focus on completing one task at a time. Breaking tasks into smaller steps makes them feel more manageable and keeps us moving forward. For example, if you need to gather supplies or organize a safe space, focus on each task one by one. Each small accomplishment boosts our confidence and reduces feelings of helplessness.

Visualization can also be a powerful tool for mental preparation. Visualization means imagining ourselves successfully handling challenges before they happen. When we mentally walk through how we would respond to an emergency, our brain starts to feel more prepared. We can practice this by picturing scenarios, like finding shelter or calming ourselves in a tense situation, and imagining the steps we would take. This practice helps us feel more comfortable and ready if those situations actually happen.

Mental and emotional preparation also means being aware of our thoughts. In high-pressure situations, negative thoughts can make us feel defeated. Practicing positive self-talk can help counteract this. Positive self-talk is when we use encouraging words with ourselves, like saying, "I can handle this" or "I am prepared." These simple statements give us a boost and help us stay motivated, even when things get tough. Practicing this daily makes it easier to rely on positive thoughts during challenging moments.

Building a strong mindset also includes preparing emotionally. Survival situations can be isolating and may involve difficult decisions, like rationing food or staying put when we want to leave. By thinking through these possibilities in advance, we can mentally prepare ourselves for the tough choices that might come. Discussing these scenarios with family members and talking openly about potential struggles helps everyone understand what to expect, reducing fear and uncertainty.

It's also valuable to connect with others who have similar preparedness goals. Being part of a community of like-minded people can offer encouragement, shared learning, and emotional support. Talking with others who have faced similar challenges can teach us new strategies and remind us that we're not alone in our efforts. This network of support boosts our morale and helps us feel more capable, even during difficult times.

Learning practical problem-solving skills is another part of building the right mindset. Problem-solving involves breaking down a situation, understanding the main issues, and coming up with possible solutions. In survival situations, thinking logically and taking things step-by-step is often more effective than rushing in or acting on impulse. Practicing problem-solving, like troubleshooting small household issues or planning small projects, strengthens our ability to approach bigger problems calmly and effectively.

Practicing gratitude can play a surprising role in developing a survival mindset. When we appreciate what we have, like shelter, food, or family, it helps us focus on the positive. In tough times, this sense of gratitude can lift our spirits and remind us of our purpose and what's worth protecting. Even in emergencies, noticing small things to be thankful for can improve our attitude and strengthen our will to endure.

Mental and emotional preparation is just as essential as any physical readiness for survival. By cultivating resilience, adaptability, and calmness, and by using tools like positive self-talk and visualization, we strengthen our ability to face emergencies with a clear mind and a hopeful heart. Practicing these skills in everyday life ensures they're ready when we need them most. With the right mindset, we're not only prepared to survive but also to handle challenges confidently and effectively, giving ourselves the best chance for a positive outcome.

CHAPTER 2

Essential Survival Skills

Core Skills: Shelter Building, Fire Making, Water Sourcing and First Aid

In any emergency situation, a few essential survival skills can make the difference between struggling and staying safe and healthy. When you're prepared to build a shelter, make a fire, find clean water, and give basic first aid, you're better equipped to handle the challenges of being without the comforts of home or help nearby. These skills are not only valuable for surviving emergencies, but they can also teach us a lot about nature and how to look after ourselves. Knowing how to use these skills is empowering and can make us feel more confident in any situation.

One of the first essential survival skills is shelter building. A shelter is crucial for protecting ourselves from harsh weather conditions like cold, rain, and heat, which can cause discomfort or even serious health issues. To make a simple shelter, start by looking for materials around you, like tree branches, leaves, and rocks. One effective shelter type is the "lean-to," which involves propping a long branch against a tree or rock to create a slanted frame. Then, lean smaller branches against this frame, covering them with leaves and grasses to help block wind and rain. Another option, if you have a tarp or even a large plastic bag, is to create a makeshift tent by tying the ends to trees or securing it with rocks. Building a shelter doesn't require fancy tools; it only requires the ability to use natural resources effectively. Remember that when choosing a location, avoid areas with water pooling, like valleys, and try to find a spot that's a little elevated and safe from wind.

Another vital skill is fire-making. Fire provides warmth, a way to cook food, and a method for purifying water. To start a fire, you need three things: tinder (tiny, dry materials like dried leaves or grass), kindling (slightly bigger sticks), and fuel (larger logs or pieces of wood). Begin by gathering these materials and stacking the tinder in a small pile at the center of your fire area. Use a lighter or matches, if you have them, to ignite the tinder, blowing on it gently to keep it going. If you don't have these tools, you can try the "fire-by-friction" method by rubbing sticks together, though this takes more practice and patience. Once the tinder is burning, slowly add the kindling, and then larger fuel logs as the fire grows. It's important to make sure your fire is built safely, away from dry leaves or branches that could catch fire accidentally. When you're done using it, be sure to put out your fire completely by pouring water on it and stirring the ashes.

Water sourcing is perhaps the most critical survival skill because we can't go without clean drinking water for very long. The first step in finding water is to look for natural sources, like rivers, lakes, or streams. However, water from these sources often isn't safe to drink right away, as it may contain bacteria or other contaminants. To make the water safe, it should be purified, and one of the best methods is boiling. Bring water to a rolling boil for at least one minute to kill most harmful germs. If boiling isn't possible, another option is using a portable water filter, which can remove many contaminants, or adding water purification tablets, which kill bacteria and viruses. In areas where no open water sources are available, you might collect rainwater or dew from plants, although these methods require careful handling to avoid contamination. Staying hydrated is essential for keeping energy levels up and avoiding dehydration.

Knowing basic first aid is essential in emergencies to treat injuries and prevent infections. Even minor injuries, if left untreated, can lead to more significant problems over time. One important aspect of first aid is wound care. If you have a cut or scrape, the first step is to clean it thoroughly with clean water to remove any dirt or debris. If you have antiseptic wipes, use them to disinfect the wound, then cover it with a bandage to keep it protected. For burns, it's best to cool the area as soon as possible by running it under cool water for several minutes, then covering it with a sterile bandage. If someone has a sprain or fracture, it's essential to keep the injured part immobilized by creating a splint, which can be done using a straight stick or piece of wood and tying it with cloth or strips of clothing.

Another aspect of first aid includes knowing how to manage dehydration and shock. Dehydration, which happens when the body loses more water than it takes in, can cause dizziness, dry mouth, and tiredness. Rehydrate by drinking small sips of clean water over time, as drinking too much too quickly can sometimes make things worse. Shock is a physical reaction to a traumatic event or injury, and it can cause symptoms like shallow breathing, cold skin, and confusion. To help someone in shock, have them lie down with their feet elevated, keep them warm, and reassure them until help arrives. Being calm and supportive is as important as the physical care you provide.

Practicing these core skills; shelter building, fire making, water sourcing, and first aid helps us feel ready and capable. While some of these techniques may take practice, they're valuable abilities that make a real difference in survival situations. Knowing how to build a simple shelter can give us a safe place to rest, starting a fire can keep us warm and cook our food, finding and purifying water keeps us hydrated, and first aid skills allow us to handle injuries safely. These essential survival skills make us more self-sufficient and prepared for whatever situations we may encounter.

Step-by-Step Guide to Mastering Critical Survival Skills

Mastering survival skills takes practice, patience, and a good understanding of the basics. Each skill has steps that make learning easier, and it's helpful to start with beginner techniques before moving to more advanced ones. Learning these skills can help anyone feel more confident and prepared, whether in the wilderness or during an emergency situation at home. Here's a breakdown of how to get good at shelter building, fire starting, water sourcing, and first aid.

For shelter building, the first step is knowing where to set up a shelter. Look for a flat, dry spot, ideally on higher ground, where there's less chance of water pooling if it rains. Make sure it's protected from strong winds, like next to a large tree or rock. Gather materials like branches, leaves, and grasses for a simple shelter. A beginner's shelter to try is the "lean-to," where you use a long branch to create a slanted frame against a tree. Stack smaller branches against this frame and cover them with leaves and grasses to make it warmer and more windproof. For a more advanced option, the "debris hut" works well in colder weather. To build one, form a structure with sticks like a small tent frame, cover it with thick layers of leaves or moss, then add more sticks on top. The thicker the layer, the better it will hold warmth. Always remember that a good shelter should keep out wind, rain, and cold, and should be safe to sleep in.

Starting a fire is another key skill, and it's useful for warmth, cooking, and water purification. The most straightforward way is to use a lighter or matches, so keep those in your emergency kit. Gather three types of materials: tinder (like dry leaves or small twigs), kindling (medium-sized sticks), and fuel (larger logs). Stack a small pile of tinder and light it, then gradually add kindling and larger logs as the fire builds up. If you don't have matches or a lighter, a fire starter like flint and steel can create sparks. Strike the flint against steel over a pile of tinder to ignite it. For a more advanced method, fire-by-friction uses two sticks, but it takes time and practice. Using a bow drill, which involves a flexible stick tied to a cord or shoelace and spun against a baseboard, is a traditional way to make fire through friction. Fire safety is essential always keep water or sand nearby to put it out, and ensure it's completely extinguished when finished.

Water sourcing and purification are crucial skills. Start by learning where to find natural water, like streams, rivers, or lakes. Collect water using a clean container and make sure to purify it before drinking. Boiling is one of the most effective methods, so if you have a metal container, boil the water for at least one minute to kill bacteria and viruses. A water filter is a helpful tool to have and can remove most contaminants, but read the instructions to understand how it works. You can also use water purification tablets, which are small and easy to carry. Drop a tablet into a liter of water, wait for the recommended time (usually around 30 minutes), and the water will be safe to drink. If you're ready for advanced skills, you can learn how to collect rainwater using a tarp to funnel it into a container, or gather dew from plants using a clean cloth in the early morning, wringing it into a container. Always remember that untreated water can carry harmful germs, so it's essential to make sure it's clean before drinking.

Knowing basic first aid is essential for treating injuries and staying healthy. Start by learning how to clean wounds, which prevents infection. Use clean water to rinse dirt and debris, and apply antiseptic if you have it, then cover the wound with a clean bandage. For burns, cool the area with water, then cover it with a sterile bandage. Having a well-stocked first aid kit makes a big difference, so try to keep items like adhesive bandages, gauze, antiseptic wipes, and pain relief medicine handy. For sprains, the "RICE" method (Rest, Ice, Compression, Elevation) can help reduce swelling and pain. Wrap the sprained area with an elastic bandage, elevate it, and rest to avoid further injury. In more advanced first aid, learning cardiopulmonary resuscitation (CPR) can save lives, especially in cases where someone's breathing or heartbeat has stopped. Taking a first aid course can help you master these techniques and give you hands-on practice.

Once you've practiced these survival skills, there are ways to build on them. In shelter building, for example, experimenting with different materials and designs can make your shelters stronger and more comfortable. For fire-making, try starting a fire in damp conditions to understand how different materials respond. With water sourcing, familiarize yourself with the local plants and environment, as this can help you identify reliable water sources more quickly. As for first aid, keeping your skills fresh with regular practice, like changing out supplies in your kit and reviewing techniques, ensures you're always ready.

Learning survival skills in small steps makes them easier to understand and apply in real situations. By breaking down each task and practicing regularly, you'll not only get better at these skills but also feel more prepared for any challenge you might face. Practicing these skills doesn't require dangerous situations; they can be practiced safely and thoughtfully. When you know how to find shelter, make fire, purify water, and give first aid, you gain independence and the ability to handle emergencies with confidence and calmness.

CHAPTER 3

Stockpiling Essentials

Must-Have Items for Your Emergency Kit

An emergency kit is like a toolbox for survival, filled with items that can help you through a range of challenging situations. Having the right supplies can make a huge difference in emergencies, providing safety, health, and comfort when you need it most. The following items are essentials for a well-rounded emergency kit, each serving a specific purpose to help you stay prepared in different scenarios.

Food and water are the top essentials. In emergencies, access to food and clean water can be limited, so it's important to have a reliable supply. Non-perishable foods are best since they don't spoil quickly, so look for canned goods, dried fruits, nuts, protein bars, and other long-lasting items. Aim to store enough food to last each person in your household for at least three days. Water is just as important; aim to store at least one gallon per person per day, enough to cover drinking and basic hygiene. Water purification tablets or a portable water filter are also smart additions, as they allow you to purify natural water sources if your stored water runs out.

First aid supplies are essential for treating injuries and managing health issues. A well-stocked first aid kit includes bandages, gauze, antiseptic wipes, adhesive tape, pain relievers, and tools like tweezers and scissors. These items help you treat cuts, scrapes, and other minor injuries on the spot, preventing infections. For more serious injuries, having items like sterile gloves and a first aid manual can be useful. If anyone in your household takes prescription medications, it's a good idea to include a small supply in your kit in case of an extended emergency.

Tools and survival gear make handling difficult situations easier. A multi-tool is incredibly useful since it combines several tools, like a knife, screwdriver, and scissors, in one compact item. A flashlight with extra batteries or a hand-crank version is also important because, in many emergencies, power outages are common. A whistle can help you signal for help if you're trapped or need to attract attention. Duct tape and sturdy rope are versatile items, helpful for repairs, creating makeshift shelters, or securing supplies. Including a good-quality map of your area, along with a compass, can help you navigate if you need to move to a safer location or find resources.

For warmth and shelter, an emergency blanket and a small, durable tarp can be lifesavers. An emergency blanket, sometimes called a "space blanket," is lightweight and retains body heat, keeping you warm if you're in a cold environment. A tarp can be used to create a simple shelter to protect you from the elements, whether it's rain, wind, or intense sun. In cold climates, consider adding extra hand warmers or layers of clothing in your kit for additional warmth.

Hygiene and sanitation items are often overlooked but can be crucial. Basic hygiene helps prevent infections and keeps you comfortable in an emergency. Include items like wet wipes, hand sanitizer, a small bar of soap, and a roll of toilet paper. If possible, add a small portable toilet or disposable bags for sanitation, especially if you live in a place where plumbing may be affected. Feminine hygiene products, toothbrushes, toothpaste, and other personal care items are also important for comfort and cleanliness.

Communication tools are vital for staying connected. A battery-powered or hand-crank radio allows you to receive updates from authorities about the emergency, which can be essential for your safety. A fully charged portable charger can keep your phone or other small electronics running, which is especially useful for contacting family or emergency services. Include extra batteries for any devices in your kit, as well as a list of important contacts in case your phone runs out of power.

Personal documents and some cash can be extremely helpful if you need to evacuate or access services. Make photocopies of identification, insurance policies, medical records, and any other important documents. Store them in a waterproof bag to keep them safe from water damage. Having some cash on hand is useful too, as Automated Teller Machine and card readers may not work if there's a power outage.

Protective gear can provide safety and comfort in certain situations. Masks, gloves, and goggles can shield you from smoke, dust, or chemicals, which might be present in natural disasters like wildfires or industrial accidents. Work gloves are helpful if you need to clear debris or handle rough materials. In some situations, it might also be useful to have a helmet for head protection.

Consider adding items for comfort and morale. Being in an emergency situation is stressful, so having small items that bring comfort or help pass the time can make a difference. Things like a deck of cards, a small notebook with a pen, or a book can help occupy your mind. Including a small supply of favorite snacks or treats can also be a morale booster.

Each item in an emergency kit has a specific role that contributes to your survival and well-being. The basics like food, water, and first aid are essential for everyone, while other items such as tools, communication devices, and hygiene supplies add versatility and help you handle different situations. Having these items packed and ready ensures that you'll have what you need to face a range of challenges confidently, whether you're sheltering at home or evacuating to a safer place.

Best Practices for Food Storage and Long-Term Shelf Life

Storing food for emergencies is all about keeping your supplies fresh, safe, and accessible. With the right techniques, you can ensure that your food remains nutritious and ready to eat when you need it most. Understanding the best practices for food storage and knowing the shelf life of different items will help you make smart decisions about what to stockpile. Rotation, storage conditions, and choosing the right foods are all essential parts of effective food storage.

One of the most important factors for food storage is the environment where you keep your supplies. Food should ideally be stored in a cool, dry, and dark place. High temperatures can speed up spoilage, so try to keep your food supplies in an area that stays around 50-70°F (10-21°C). Light can also cause food to deteriorate, which is why it's best to store food in opaque containers or in a dark area. Humidity is another big factor to watch. Too much moisture can cause mold, rust, and spoilage, so it's helpful to store food in airtight, moisture-proof containers to protect it from humidity.

Selecting the right foods for storage can make a big difference in how long your supplies last. Non-perishable items are ideal since they have longer shelf lives and don't require refrigeration. Foods like rice, pasta, beans, lentils, oats, canned meats, dried fruits, nuts, and powdered milk are excellent choices because they are shelf-stable and provide essential nutrients. These foods can last for years if stored properly. Canned goods are also a great option since they are sealed to prevent spoilage and typically have a shelf life of two to five years, sometimes even longer.

Understanding the shelf life of different foods is helpful so you know how long you can keep each item. Foods like white rice, pasta, and dried beans can last up to 30 years if they're stored properly in airtight containers with oxygen absorbers. Canned foods usually last between two to five years, depending on the type, although high-acid foods like tomatoes and citrus might have a shorter shelf life. Grains, nuts, and seeds can also be stored long-term, but they may need to be kept in the freezer if you're planning to store them for over a year, as their natural oils can go rancid over time.

One of the most effective ways to ensure you always have fresh food in your stockpile is through rotation. Rotation means using the oldest food first and replenishing it with new stock. This way, your food supply is continuously cycled, reducing the chance of spoilage. To make this easier, label each item with its purchase or expiry date. Then, when you add new food, place it behind the older stock, so you're always using the oldest items first. This approach not only keeps your supplies fresh but also makes it easier to monitor what you have.

Packaging also plays a crucial role in extending food shelf life. Using airtight containers, vacuum-sealed bags, or Mylar bags with oxygen absorbers helps reduce exposure to air, which can cause food to spoil. Mylar bags are particularly useful for storing dry goods like rice, pasta, and beans, as they offer a strong barrier against light, moisture, and oxygen. Oxygen absorbers are small packets that remove oxygen from the packaging, creating an environment that's less likely to support bacteria and mold growth, which keeps your food fresher for longer.

Another consideration is whether to keep certain foods in their original packaging or transfer them to other containers. For items that come in thin plastic or cardboard, it's often better to transfer them into more durable, airtight containers. For instance, storing grains, flour, and sugar in food-grade buckets with lids helps protect them from pests and moisture. Glass jars, metal cans, and heavy-duty plastic containers are all great options for food storage, as they are sturdy and provide an effective barrier.

In addition to packaging, certain preservation methods can also help extend shelf life. Dehydrating and freeze-drying are two popular methods for long-term food storage. Dehydrating removes moisture from food, making it lightweight and shelf-stable, while freeze-drying locks in nutrients and flavor. Many companies offer freeze-dried fruits, vegetables, and even full meals that can last 25 years or more. While these foods might be more expensive upfront, they're a convenient option for long-term storage and are often easy to prepare by simply adding water.

To make sure you're storing a well-rounded diet, aim for a balance of carbohydrates, proteins, fats, vitamins, and minerals. Carbohydrate-rich foods like rice and pasta provide energy, while canned meats, beans, and lentils are good protein sources.

Nuts, seeds, and oils are important for fats, which are essential for absorbing certain vitamins and keeping you satisfied. Dried fruits and vegetables can add vitamins and fiber to your diet, and you can also consider multivitamins as a supplement in case fresh foods are unavailable.

It's important to inspect your food supplies regularly. Every few months, go through your stockpile to check for signs of spoilage, rust on cans, or broken seals. If you notice any unusual smells, discoloration, or damaged packaging, discard the item to prevent contamination. Regular checks help ensure that your supplies are safe to consume and allow you to restock any items that may be running low.

Successful food storage for emergencies involves understanding ideal storage conditions, choosing long-lasting foods, practicing rotation, and using proper packaging. By following these best practices, you can create a reliable, nutritious stockpile that supports your health and well-being in any emergency. Not only does this approach help protect your food from spoilage, but it also provides peace of mind knowing you're prepared for unexpected situations.

Essential Tools and Equipment for Every Emergency

In an emergency, having the right tools and equipment can make all the difference in keeping yourself and your family safe, comfortable, and well-prepared. This section explains essential tools that every prepper should have, from basic survival gear to specialized equipment. Knowing what to include in your toolkit and how to store it properly can help you face a variety of situations with confidence.

One of the most versatile tools for emergencies is a multi-tool. These compact devices combine several tools into one, including a knife, pliers, screwdriver, scissors, and more. A quality multi-tool can handle a wide range of tasks, like cutting materials, tightening screws, or even helping with basic repairs. It's useful for everyday tasks, too, and can save you space and weight in your emergency bag.

A reliable knife is essential. A fixed-blade knife, especially one with a sturdy, full tang (meaning the blade runs through the entire handle), is better for tough jobs than folding knives. This tool is useful for preparing food, cutting rope, or even carving wood if you need to build a shelter. Choose a knife that's comfortable to hold, durable, and easy to sharpen. A folding knife or pocket knife is also handy for lighter tasks and can be easily carried in your pocket or bag.

A fire-starting tool is another must-have item. Matches and lighters are the simplest tools, but waterproof or stormproof matches are even better because they can withstand wet or windy conditions. In addition, a fire steel (or ferro rod) is a long-lasting tool that can create sparks even in damp conditions. Fire starters are essential for warmth, cooking, and signaling in emergencies, so it's wise to have a few different options available.

Flashlights and headlamps are essential for visibility in low light or dark environments. A headlamp is especially useful because it allows you to keep your hands free while you work. When choosing a flashlight, look for one with a long battery life and multiple brightness settings. Consider adding a solar-powered or hand-crank flashlight so you're not dependent on batteries alone. It's also helpful to pack extra batteries in a safe, dry place to ensure they're ready when needed.

Shelter-building tools, like a compact folding shovel or a small hatchet, can help you create shelter and clear areas for camp. A folding shovel is ideal for digging fire pits or even creating emergency latrines. A hatchet can be used for chopping wood for fires or building makeshift structures. Both tools should be lightweight yet strong enough to handle rough outdoor tasks.

Paracord, or parachute cord, is another essential item. This lightweight, strong rope has countless uses, from tying down tarps for shelter to creating makeshift handles or even repairing broken gear. Paracord can also be unraveled into smaller strands to use as fishing line or thread. It's versatile, easy to carry, and can hold significant weight.

A first aid kit is critical for treating injuries and keeping you healthy in emergencies. Your kit should include bandages, antiseptics, tweezers, pain relievers, and any medications specific to your needs. For preppers, it's beneficial to have additional supplies like a tourniquet, gauze, and even a first aid manual. Proper first aid can prevent minor injuries from becoming serious and can make a big difference in survival situations.

Navigation tools, like a compass and map, are valuable if you need to travel on foot without GPS. While smartphones have built-in GPS, they rely on battery power and network coverage, which can be unreliable in emergencies. A simple compass and a paper map of your area can guide you if you need to find your way without electronic devices.

Water filtration and purification gear is necessary for staying hydrated, especially if you're in the wilderness. Portable water filters, such as a straw filter or pump filter, allow you to drink from natural water sources by removing harmful bacteria and parasites. Water purification tablets are also useful for treating larger quantities of water. Keeping a portable water filter or a few purification tablets in your emergency kit can help you access safe drinking water wherever you are.

For communication, a battery-powered or hand-crank radio is essential. An emergency radio can provide updates on weather, news, and rescue operations. Some emergency radios come with built-in flashlights, solar panels, and even USB chargers for your phone. A hand-crank option ensures that you have access to critical information even if you run out of batteries.

A survival blanket, also known as a space blanket, is a lightweight, heat-reflective blanket that helps keep you warm. It's compact and can fit easily in your kit but provides significant warmth by reflecting body heat back to you. This is especially important if you're in a cold environment and need to maintain body temperature.

Storage is important to ensure your gear is organized, accessible, and protected. A sturdy backpack with multiple compartments can help you keep tools, food, and supplies well-organized. Consider using waterproof bags or containers for items sensitive to moisture, like fire-starting tools and first aid supplies. Being organized saves time and stress in emergencies, so make sure you know where each item is in your kit.

Protective gear, such as gloves and sturdy boots, is also essential, especially for situations where you'll be handling heavy objects, working with sharp tools, or walking through rough terrain. Gloves protect your hands from blisters, cuts, and cold, while boots provide support and protection for your feet. Durable, comfortable clothing that suits the climate of your area is also important.

Self-defense tools are worth considering based on the environment you're preparing for. Pepper spray, a whistle, or a small personal alarm can provide a sense of security. These tools are meant to deter threats or attract attention if you're in trouble.

Having these essential tools and equipment stored correctly and accessible means you're more prepared to handle emergencies calmly and effectively. Whether it's building a shelter, staying warm, treating an injury, or finding your way, each tool serves a specific purpose that supports your well-being and safety. Preparing your emergency kit with care can make a huge difference in staying safe and resilient in challenging situations.

CHAPTER 4

Home Security and Defense

Securing Your Home Against Potential Threats

Securing your home against potential threats is essential for safety and peace of mind, especially in emergency situations when risks can increase. By strengthening key areas around your home, setting up physical barriers, and reinforcing entry points, you can make your home a safer place. This section covers some basic strategies for identifying and securing weak points, reinforcing doors and windows, and establishing a secure perimeter to keep potential intruders at bay.

The first step to a secure home is to assess its weak points. Walk around the outside of your home and carefully examine areas that could allow easy access. These often include doors, windows, the garage, and other entry points. Think like an intruder and look for places where they might try to break in. Fences, hedges, or tall plants near windows can give a hiding place to potential threats, so consider trimming any vegetation around your home. A clear, well-lit exterior makes it harder for anyone to sneak up unnoticed.

Doors are one of the most important parts of home security. Reinforcing doors, especially exterior ones, can help make your home more resistant to forced entry. Solid-core doors, made from materials like wood or metal, are generally stronger than hollow-core doors. Make sure your door frames are sturdy as well, as a weak frame can be an easy point for intruders to break through. Installing a deadbolt is another essential step, as this type of lock adds an extra layer of security compared to standard door locks. You can also reinforce the area where the deadbolt is placed by using longer screws, which make it much harder to force open.

Windows are another key area to secure. If possible, consider installing impact-resistant glass or window security film, which makes it harder for the glass to break. For windows that open, install window locks or bars to add an extra level of protection. Sliding windows or doors are particularly vulnerable, so placing a metal rod or dowel in the track can prevent them from being opened from the outside. Closing blinds or curtains at night also helps reduce visibility into your home, which discourages potential intruders from seeing valuables inside.

Creating a secure perimeter around your property helps deter potential threats before they even reach your doors or windows. Fencing is one way to establish a clear boundary. Strong, tall fences are harder to climb, especially if they have pointed tops or smooth surfaces. Gates should be securely locked, and regular checks for any damage to fences or gates are important for keeping your perimeter strong. If you live in an area prone to wildlife intrusions, fencing can also help keep animals out.

Lighting is another powerful security measure. Installing motion-activated lights around your home can startle intruders and prevent them from approaching undetected. Lights near entry points like doors, windows, and garages help you see any unusual activity and can also signal to passersby that your home is being monitored. Solar-powered lights are convenient as they don't require wiring and will continue to work even during power outages.

In addition to physical barriers, technology can enhance home security. Security cameras provide a watchful eye on key areas of your home. Today's cameras are compact, affordable, and easy to set up, and many can be accessed from your smartphone. Consider placing cameras at entry points and high-traffic areas to monitor any unusual activity. A doorbell camera, for example, allows you to see who's at the door even if you're not home, giving you peace of mind and a record of visitors.

Alarm systems are also effective for alerting you to break-ins. Basic alarms sound if a door or window is opened while the system is armed, but more advanced systems can send alerts directly to your phone or notify a security company. Even a simple alarm can be a strong deterrent for intruders. Some alarms also offer features like window sensors, glass break detectors, and panic buttons, which can quickly alert you in an emergency.

Establishing a security routine is equally important. Checking that doors and windows are locked each night and when leaving the house can prevent many potential break-ins. Reinforce these routines with family members so that everyone knows how to keep the home secure. If you plan to be away for an extended period, ask a trusted neighbor or friend to check on your home and pick up any mail or packages, as accumulated items can signal to others that the house is empty.

In addition to these measures, it's wise to have a plan for different scenarios. Know how to respond if you suspect someone is attempting to enter your home, and have an emergency contact list easily accessible. Teaching children basic security practices, like not opening the door for strangers or knowing emergency phone numbers, adds an extra layer of preparedness for everyone in the household.

Securing your home is a combination of physical preparation and creating habits that reinforce safety. By assessing your home's weak points, strengthening entryways, setting up a secure perimeter, and using technology to your advantage, you can create a strong defense against potential intruders. While no plan can guarantee complete protection, taking these steps can significantly reduce risks and improve your family's safety. Being proactive and aware of your surroundings are key to staying one step ahead and ensuring that your home remains a safe haven, no matter the situation outside.

Self-Defense Strategies and Combat Skills for Preppers

Self-defense skills are essential for staying safe in uncertain situations. For preppers, learning practical strategies for self-defense can help build confidence and provide critical protection. This involves understanding basic combat techniques, knowing how to protect yourself if faced with a weapon, and learning how to use everyday items as improvised tools for defense. Each of these skills is about using your mind, body, and available resources effectively, rather than just physical strength. Staying alert and assessing threats are also key parts of self-defense that help you avoid danger when possible.

Hand-to-hand combat focuses on using your body to protect yourself if confronted by someone threatening. One of the most important parts of self-defense is learning how to stand and move. The "ready stance" is an effective way to position yourself: keep your feet shoulder-width apart, knees slightly bent, with one foot slightly behind the other. This stance helps you stay balanced and able to move quickly if needed. Raising your hands to about chest height in a relaxed manner allows you to protect your face while signaling you want to avoid conflict. Practicing this stance is simple but valuable because it gives you stability and keeps you ready for any situation.

A key part of self-defense is knowing where to aim in order to maximize impact with minimal force. In a threatening situation, aim for sensitive areas that will disable the attacker quickly, such as the eyes, nose, throat, or knees. For example, a quick strike to the nose with the heel of your hand can be enough to create an opportunity to escape. Simple moves, like kicking the knee, can cause someone to lose balance, making it easier to get away. Remember, the goal isn't to fight longer than needed but to find an opening to escape safely.

If the attacker grabs you, learning basic escape techniques can be highly effective. For instance, if someone grabs your wrist, you can often break free by twisting your wrist towards the attacker's thumb, which is usually the weakest point in their grip. Practicing these simple escapes helps prepare you to respond quickly. You don't need to overpower the attacker; instead, focus on using leverage to break free.

Another critical aspect of self-defense is defending yourself if a weapon is involved. If possible, prioritize distance; weapons pose the greatest threat when they're close. If you can create space, it's often safer. However, if escape is not possible, be aware of the weapon's reach and try to disrupt the attacker's control of it. For example, if faced with a knife, try to use a solid object nearby (like a chair or bag) to put a barrier between you and the attacker.

Always aim to disarm only as a last resort, as trying to control a weapon can be very risky.

Improvised tools can offer valuable protection when you don't have self-defense gear. Everyday items such as a pen, flashlight, or even a set of keys can serve as tools to protect yourself. A pen can be used to strike sensitive areas, like the neck, while keys held between your fingers can help create a strong defense. These objects give you an advantage, as they allow you to focus force in a smaller area and increase the impact of your movements. Practicing how to use these items safely and effectively is essential; it's about using them to distract or incapacitate an attacker just enough to allow for an escape.

Situational awareness is another essential skill. This involves staying alert to your surroundings and recognizing potential dangers before they escalate. Knowing how to assess threats is critical for preppers. For example, if you sense someone is following you, make an immediate plan for a safe exit. Try to move towards well-lit, populated areas if possible, and avoid isolated spots. Being aware of exits, keeping a clear path in mind, and spotting places where you can seek help (like a store or other public area) are all ways to maintain control in a situation. Practicing these skills in daily life can help make awareness second nature.

Staying calm in high-pressure situations is also a crucial part of self-defense. Practicing deep breathing exercises can help control fear, allowing you to think more clearly. A steady mind is often your best asset, as fear can hinder your ability to act effectively. By training yourself to focus on breathing in and out slowly, you can manage stress and remain focused on the situation, which helps you think through your response. Remember, mental preparation is as important as physical skills.

In addition to these techniques, setting boundaries can often help prevent situations from escalating.

For instance, using a strong voice to say something like, "Stop! Don't come any closer," can be effective in discouraging someone who might be approaching you. Confidence in your voice can send a message that you are not an easy target, often causing potential attackers to think twice. Setting boundaries also reinforces your own sense of control, reminding you that you are capable of defending yourself if needed.

Regular practice is key to becoming proficient in self-defense. Many of these techniques are simple, but muscle memory is important for them to be effective in real situations. Consider practicing with a friend or taking a self-defense class. Training under the guidance of an instructor can provide hands-on experience and valuable feedback. Learning from a professional also helps ensure that you're using techniques safely and effectively.

Self-defense is about protecting yourself by using a combination of physical skills, awareness, and confidence. Practicing hand-to-hand techniques, knowing how to handle threats with weapons, and using everyday objects as improvised tools can greatly enhance your ability to stay safe. Cultivating awareness and calmness under pressure, setting strong boundaries, and reinforcing these habits through regular practice make self-defense a practical and empowering skill for preppers. By mastering these strategies, you build resilience and readiness for handling any situation confidently and with control.

Enhancing Security with Alarm Systems and Surveillance

Enhancing home security with alarm systems, surveillance cameras, and motion detectors plays a crucial role in creating a safer living environment. In emergency situations or times of uncertainty, these tools help protect people and property, giving a sense of control and peace of mind. Alarm systems, surveillance technology, and motion detection each serve unique purposes, but when combined, they form a comprehensive security network that can alert you to potential threats and deter intruders.

Alarm systems are one of the most widely used and effective forms of security. They're designed to detect unauthorized entry and sound a loud alarm that alerts you, your neighbors, or a monitoring center. This immediate response can scare off intruders before they even have a chance to do any harm. Alarms can be customized to suit various needs; for instance, some systems can be set to detect not only entry through doors and windows but also forced entry attempts or glass breaking. Many alarm systems are connected to smartphone apps, allowing you to monitor your home remotely, control the system, and receive alerts in real-time if something triggers it. This remote monitoring can be especially helpful during an emergency or if you need to leave your property unattended for an extended period.

Surveillance cameras add another important layer to home security. Cameras provide visual monitoring, capturing footage of all activities in and around your home. Some cameras are highly advanced, offering features like night vision, two-way audio, and high-definition video quality. Positioning cameras at key points; such as entry doors, pathways, and any secluded areas gives you a better view of potential threats. Surveillance footage also helps in identifying intruders if an incident does occur, which can be valuable for reporting to law enforcement or identifying suspicious behavior early on. Additionally, modern security cameras often have motion detection and can send instant notifications when they sense movement. This allows you to assess potential threats quickly and respond appropriately.

Motion detectors are another essential security feature that enhances your home's defense. These sensors detect any movement within their range, triggering alarms or cameras to capture activity.

Motion detectors are typically installed in rooms, hallways, and outside near doors or gates to catch anyone attempting to enter undetected. Some motion detectors are even smart enough to distinguish between different types of movement, helping to avoid false alarms from pets or swaying branches. A properly placed motion detector will cover any gaps in your security system, making it more difficult for intruders to find a way in unnoticed. Some models include infrared technology, which detects body heat, allowing them to work effectively even in low light or complete darkness.

Choosing the right security technology depends on your specific needs and budget, but many systems today offer options that make it easy to tailor protection. For example, a combination of basic alarms with a few outdoor cameras might work well for small homes, while larger properties might benefit from multiple cameras, advanced motion detectors, and a centralized alarm system. When selecting equipment, it's essential to consider factors such as weather resistance for outdoor devices, battery life, and whether the technology requires professional installation or can be set up independently. Many systems are designed to be user-friendly, with simple setup and maintenance requirements, making them accessible even for those without a lot of technical expertise.

A well-planned security system also includes monitoring services, which allow a security company to respond to alerts. These services work by notifying a monitoring center if an alarm is triggered, and the center will contact you or emergency services if necessary. Monitoring provides an extra layer of security, as someone is always available to respond if an incident occurs. This can be particularly valuable if you're away from home or unable to check your security system yourself. Some security companies offer packages that include monitoring for fire, smoke, and carbon monoxide, adding to overall home safety.

Technology integration in modern security systems makes it easier to monitor and control every aspect of your home security from a smartphone or computer. For instance, many systems now work with smart home devices, like voice-activated assistants, allowing you to control alarms and cameras hands-free. Some systems even use artificial intelligence to analyze video feeds for unusual behavior, sending alerts if something seems suspicious. Smart home integration allows for customized security settings, giving you greater control over which areas are monitored at what times, and allowing easy adjustments as your security needs change.

In addition to deterring intruders, security systems play an essential role during emergencies like natural disasters or unexpected evacuations. For example, smoke and carbon monoxide detectors connected to your alarm system can alert you to fires or hazardous gases, potentially saving lives by providing early warnings. Surveillance footage can also be valuable for documenting any damage caused by natural disasters, aiding in insurance claims and recovery efforts. A reliable security system helps you prepare for and respond to various types of emergencies, reducing the chance of losses or injuries.

The visible presence of security measures like cameras and alarms can act as a strong deterrent to would-be intruders. Studies have shown that homes with security systems are significantly less likely to be targeted by burglars. When someone sees a camera or an alarm system in place, they are often discouraged from attempting to enter. Clearly displaying signs that indicate a monitored alarm or surveillance system can further enhance this effect, making it clear that any attempt to break in will not go unnoticed.

Regular maintenance of security equipment is also essential for it to work effectively. Periodically check your cameras, alarms, and motion detectors to ensure they are fully functional. Replace batteries as needed and verify that all devices remain connected to their respective control panels or apps. Testing the system occasionally helps identify any weak points or malfunctions before they compromise security. Many security systems have self-testing features or will send alerts if they detect a problem, making it easier to keep everything running smoothly.

Alarm systems, surveillance cameras, and motion detectors offer strong security that helps protect your home in various situations. Each element adds value, and when combined, they create a comprehensive system that is difficult for intruders to bypass. Modern technology offers flexibility in how you set up and monitor these systems, whether through a professional service or with Do It Yourself options. By using these tools and following best practices, you can create a safer environment, stay prepared for emergencies, and enjoy greater peace of mind knowing that your home and loved ones are well-protected.

CHAPTER 5

Communication and Information

Why Communication is Key in Crisis Situations

Communication plays a crucial role in survival during a crisis, and it affects nearly every aspect of how people respond to emergencies. Whether it's a natural disaster, an unexpected accident, or a prolonged period of social unrest, effective communication can mean the difference between confusion and clear decision-making, isolation and coordinated effort, and even survival or serious harm. Understanding why communication is so essential in these situations helps individuals and groups make better preparations and develop the skills they need to face crises with confidence.

One of the most important functions of communication in an emergency is enabling quick and effective decision-making. During a crisis, time is often limited, and the choices made in those initial moments can greatly influence the outcome. By staying connected, people can quickly gather the information they need to assess their situation, understand the risks, and decide on the best course of action. For example, receiving real-time updates from weather authorities during a storm or wildfire can help families decide when it's safest to evacuate, where to go, and what route to take. Without clear and up-to-date information, people may feel uncertain or panic, making decisions that could put them at risk.

Communication also plays a key role in coordination, which is vital when working with others to achieve a common goal. In an emergency, family members, neighbors, and even strangers often have to rely on each other to get through challenging situations. Good communication helps people divide tasks, understand each other's needs, and support each other in practical ways. For instance, in an extended power outage, families might need to share resources, such as water and food, or work together to repair damaged property. Being able to clearly communicate plans, responsibilities, and updates helps everyone work more effectively and prevents misunderstandings that could lead to frustration or conflict.

Another essential function of communication in crisis situations is maintaining morale. Crises can be emotionally taxing, causing stress, fear, and sometimes despair. Staying in touch with loved ones, friends, or support networks provides encouragement, reassurance, and a sense of community, which helps people stay calm and focused. In survival situations, morale can significantly impact one's resilience, affecting the ability to persevere and stay positive. Simple check-ins, words of support, and sharing small victories can uplift spirits and create a sense of unity. People feel stronger and more capable when they know they aren't facing challenges alone.

The role of communication extends beyond immediate needs and also affects long-term survival efforts. For instance, during an ongoing crisis, staying informed about resources, updates from authorities, or health advisories is critical for adapting to changing conditions. Information about local resources, such as food or medical aid distributions, can prevent shortages and ensure people know where to find help when they need it. Without reliable communication, people may miss these essential updates, making it harder to meet basic needs and increasing the risks to their safety.

Communication tools and methods can vary depending on the situation. In some cases, people might have access to their usual devices, like smartphones, tablets, or computers. These devices allow for a wide range of communication options, such as calling, texting, or using social media to send messages and receive news. However, in situations where power or networks are disrupted, having alternative tools is essential. For example, two-way radios, walkie-talkies, and CB radios allow people to communicate over short and medium distances without relying on cell towers or internet access. Satellite phones are another useful tool, as they can function in remote areas and aren't dependent on local network infrastructure. Knowing which tools to use and how to operate them helps ensure that people stay connected no matter the conditions.

Another factor in crisis communication is ensuring messages are clear, concise, and accurate. In high-stress situations, confusion can quickly arise, and misunderstandings can lead to poor decisions. For example, if someone is guiding another person on how to reach a safe location, clear directions are necessary to prevent misinterpretations. Using simple language, verifying information before sharing it, and avoiding spreading unconfirmed rumors can all help maintain clarity. Being mindful of tone is also essential; messages should aim to inform and reassure rather than amplify fear or stress.

Learning and practicing basic communication protocols can improve readiness. For instance, families can establish a simple emergency communication plan, which may include setting up a meeting spot if they get separated, designating someone outside the immediate area as a contact person, and sharing a list of essential phone numbers. By planning these details ahead of time, families can reduce confusion if regular communication channels become unreliable. In community settings, neighbors can agree on signals or codes to communicate key information, such as needing help or confirming safety, without speaking directly.

Another way to prepare for effective communication during a crisis is to practice listening as much as speaking. Listening skills ensure that messages are correctly received and understood, avoiding repeated instructions or misunderstandings. Active listening can make a big difference when coordinating with others under pressure, as it helps each person feel respected and ensures that everyone is on the same page. In emergencies, clear communication often relies on cooperation and patience, where everyone contributes to a safe and effective response.

Respect for privacy and boundaries is also part of effective crisis communication. In stressful times, emotions can run high, and people may feel overwhelmed or sensitive. Recognizing that everyone processes situations differently, and respecting each person's needs, helps create a supportive environment. For example, some people might prefer brief check-ins rather than constant updates, while others may find comfort in more frequent contact. Respecting these differences fosters harmony and reduces unnecessary tension.

Maintaining access to reliable information sources is vital as well. Trusted sources, such as local emergency management agencies, government websites, or weather apps, provide accurate, verified information that can guide decisions. Relying on official channels reduces the risk of misinformation, which can be common in times of crisis. People should be cautious about unverified messages or sensationalized news, as these can spread quickly and create unnecessary panic.

Communication is essential in emergencies because it aids decision-making, enhances coordination, and boosts morale. It also keeps people connected to valuable information, resources, and each other. Having the right tools, practicing clear and respectful communication, and staying informed through reliable sources can significantly improve outcomes during crises. Preparing communication strategies in advance can provide peace of mind and help everyone respond to challenges with confidence and unity.

Effective Communication Methods for Preppers

Communication is one of the most powerful tools in an emergency, and having various methods at your disposal can make a big difference in safety, coordination, and peace of mind. There are many ways preppers can stay connected, from traditional devices like radios to modern apps and satellite phones. Each method has its own strengths and weaknesses, depending on the situation, so understanding these options helps preppers choose the best tools for their needs.

One of the most reliable communication tools for emergencies is the traditional two-way radio. Two-way radios are portable devices that allow users to communicate over short to medium distances without needing a cellular network or internet connection. This makes them especially useful in natural disasters, power outages, or areas with poor cell coverage. They're easy to use and widely available, often coming with multiple channels to avoid interference. The main limitation is that the range can be limited, typically only covering a few miles in urban areas, though this range extends in open areas without many obstacles. Still, two-way radios are affordable and don't require complex setup, making them a practical option for most families or groups.

For longer-range communication, CB (Citizen Band) radios offer another layer of reliability. CB radios work over greater distances than standard two-way radios, reaching up to 10-20 miles depending on terrain. They are commonly used by truck drivers but can be useful for preppers as well, especially when traveling or in isolated areas. CB radios can help users get updates from other travelers or local emergency broadcasts if internet or cellular connections are unavailable. However, they tend to be bulkier and may require more power than basic two-way radios. CB radios are great for car-to-car communication or connecting with people nearby during widespread emergencies.

Ham (amateur) radio is a powerful tool with a large range and is highly valued among serious preppers. Ham radio allows users to reach people hundreds or even thousands of miles away, depending on the equipment and weather conditions. Many ham radio operators are part of established networks that provide news, weather updates, and emergency assistance during crises. Using a ham radio requires a license, but learning to use it can be incredibly valuable for those who want to be fully prepared. Ham radio equipment can be expensive, and the setup might feel a bit complex at first. However, it's one of the most versatile options available for those committed to mastering it.

Satellite phones are another excellent tool, especially for extreme situations. Unlike radios that depend on radio waves or cell towers, satellite phones connect directly to satellites orbiting the earth. This means they work in almost any location, from dense forests to remote deserts. Satellite phones allow users to make voice calls, send texts, and even access limited internet in some cases, making them invaluable for those in very isolated regions or areas impacted by severe disasters. However, satellite phones are quite costly, both to purchase and use, as they require a subscription. They're not the most budget-friendly choice but are a reliable backup for people who prioritize communication during major crises.

Modern technology has also introduced emergency apps and messaging platforms that preppers can use when cell service and internet are still functional. For example, apps like Zello turn your phone into a walkie-talkie, allowing for push-to-talk communication over Wi-Fi or mobile data. Other apps, like Signal, WhatsApp, and Telegram, enable encrypted messaging, which can be useful for secure communications. These apps are easy to use and allow instant sharing of text, images, and location pins. However, they rely on the availability of data networks or Wi-Fi, which may not be accessible during widespread outages. For preppers, these apps are great for early-stage emergencies when services are still intact but aren't reliable for severe, prolonged crises.

Social media platforms like Twitter and Facebook can be helpful for getting real-time updates from local authorities, emergency services, and other preppers. Many government agencies now post updates on social media, so it's a good way to stay informed about weather conditions, road closures, and shelter locations. Social media also allows people to quickly connect with family and friends, sharing safety statuses and important information. However, social media can sometimes spread misinformation during crises, so it's important to verify information before acting on it. Additionally, like messaging apps, social media platforms require internet access, which may be compromised during major events.

For groups or families who need an organized way to communicate, preppers can create a communication plan that incorporates several methods. For example, they might set up a primary communication method, such as an app, but also have backup tools like two-way radios or a satellite phone if networks go down. In any crisis, having a structured plan that everyone understands reduces confusion and ensures everyone knows how to stay connected. This is especially important in situations where loved ones might be separated, such as during evacuations.

Another method to enhance communication in emergencies is by setting up emergency codes or signals. For instance, families might develop a set of code words that represent specific actions or needs, like "all clear" or "danger." Hand signals or visible markers, such as a colored flag or light, can also be useful in situations where speaking isn't possible, such as when someone is far away but within line of sight. These codes make it easier to communicate quickly and discreetly.

Some preppers choose to invest in solar chargers or hand-crank power banks to ensure their communication tools stay functional. Portable chargers provide backup power for devices like phones, radios, or satellite devices when electricity is unavailable. Solar chargers work well in sunny conditions, while hand-crank options ensure power is available regardless of the weather. Having these power sources on hand allows preppers to keep their devices operational, even during extended outages.

Communication during a crisis is not just about having the right tools; it's also about knowing how to use them effectively. Preppers can practice using these devices, ensuring everyone in the family is comfortable operating them. Regular practice helps build confidence and ensures that, in an emergency, everyone can use the tools without added stress. Learning basic troubleshooting techniques, such as checking batteries or adjusting settings, can also help in situations where time is of the essence.

Each communication method has unique advantages and limitations, so having a mix of tools allows preppers to adapt based on the type and severity of the crisis. Traditional methods like two-way radios and CB radios are great for short-distance communication, while ham radios and satellite phones cover long distances. Modern apps and social media work well when networks are functioning, while backup power sources and practiced protocols keep everything running smoothly. Preparing with multiple methods and practicing their use ensures a well-rounded approach, giving preppers confidence in their ability to stay connected in any situation.

Collecting and Analyzing Information to Stay Informed

In an emergency, having reliable information can be just as important as having food, water, or shelter. Information keeps people aware of dangers, helps them make informed decisions, and reduces fear and confusion. For preppers, knowing how to collect and analyze information is a key survival skill that can keep them and their families safe. By gathering updates from various sources and learning how to interpret them correctly, preppers can better understand what's happening and how best to respond.

To begin gathering information, preppers need to know where to look for accurate updates. Traditional sources, like local radio and television news, are among the first places to turn in a crisis. Radio stations, especially public ones, often continue broadcasting important updates even when other systems fail. A battery-operated or hand-crank radio is valuable in these situations, especially since it doesn't rely on electricity or an internet connection. Many radios have emergency alert functions to receive immediate weather and safety information from official sources.

Weather conditions can be critical to monitor in emergencies, especially in natural disasters. Preppers can access weather updates not only from traditional broadcasts but also from apps and websites like the National Weather Service (NWS) or local meteorological services. Many weather apps provide real-time radar images, warnings, and storm tracking, allowing users to see changes as they happen. While this is a convenient way to stay informed, it's important to remember that internet or mobile networks may go down during severe storms. Having a backup, such as a NOAA weather radio, ensures you still have access to alerts if other systems are interrupted.

Online platforms are another rich source of information. Social media, news websites, and government pages can provide updates and alerts in real time. Platforms like Twitter or Facebook are often used by emergency agencies to post live information on evacuations, road closures, and weather alerts. Social media can be helpful in keeping tabs on specific areas, especially for events that move quickly, such as wildfires. However, users must be careful, as social media can sometimes spread rumors or unverified reports that cause unnecessary worry. Cross-checking facts from multiple sources or official accounts, like city or national emergency management pages, helps ensure the information is accurate.

Preppers should also be familiar with emergency apps that are designed for crisis situations. Many countries have apps that provide real-time alerts and updates for natural disasters or emergency situations. For example, FEMA in the United States has an app that sends alerts for natural hazards, like floods and tornadoes, along with safety tips and shelter information. Apps like these offer a reliable source of direct information from official channels, helping users make safer, faster decisions. Keeping these apps downloaded and regularly checking for updates ensures they work correctly when needed.

In addition to staying connected to information sources, preppers should know how to analyze the information they receive. This means not only gathering information but understanding what it means for their safety and plans. For example, if a weather report indicates a coming storm, preppers should consider factors like the expected severity, timing, and likely impact on local areas. By examining different elements, preppers can decide if they need to evacuate, reinforce their shelter, or gather specific supplies.

Cross-referencing is an essential skill in analyzing information during emergencies. By comparing details from different sources, preppers get a clearer picture and can identify inconsistencies or overreactions. For instance, if one news source suggests that a nearby fire might reach a community, checking other sources, such as the local fire department's updates, can confirm whether this is a high-risk situation or an unlikely possibility. This helps avoid unnecessary panic and prepares preppers to take only the steps that are actually needed.

In situations where news is chaotic or there are conflicting reports, it's essential to stay calm and process information carefully. Panic can lead to hasty decisions or missed details, both of which can be risky. One helpful technique is to follow the 10-second rule: take a deep breath and give yourself a moment to think before acting on new information. Reviewing your preparedness plan and checking it against new updates can also keep you focused on what truly matters instead of getting overwhelmed by every small update.

Sometimes, local networks and power sources may be down, cutting off regular information channels. In these cases, preppers can turn to other, less conventional sources to stay informed. Community resources, like ham radio operators, are often valuable during disasters. Ham radio enthusiasts regularly broadcast news updates and emergency information, sometimes over long distances, making them a valuable resource when mainstream options aren't available. Some ham radio operators even organize to provide emergency response information, coordinating with local governments to share critical details with the public.

Preppers can also rely on neighbors or other members of their community to exchange information. Setting up a neighborhood communication plan beforehand allows families to check in on one another, share updates, and help each other with supplies or shelter if needed. Knowing who to turn to within your immediate surroundings can be reassuring, and sharing responsibilities lessens the pressure on any single person to monitor every news source.

To keep track of critical updates, preppers can also create a system for organizing information as it arrives. Using a notebook or a whiteboard allows for jotting down the time, source, and main points of each update. This organization is particularly helpful in fast-paced situations, like a wildfire approaching a community, where preppers need to assess how quickly events are developing and what actions are best. Writing things down ensures no detail is missed or forgotten in the rush, and reviewing past notes can offer a sense of how the situation has evolved over time.

Preppers should also be prepared for longer-term crises, where staying informed over days or weeks might be necessary. In these scenarios, information about food and water sources, medical facilities, or transportation routes becomes more relevant. Preppers should track these details along with immediate safety updates. They might consider designating family members to focus on different types of information, such as one person for news and another for weather, ensuring everyone has a manageable role.

In any emergency, being informed is key, but so is focusing on what matters most. Prioritizing information that impacts immediate safety, such as evacuation orders or severe weather changes, is crucial. Less urgent updates, like general news or minor event developments, can be noted but don't require immediate action. This prioritization helps preppers manage their attention and energy, especially in situations that last for extended periods.

The ability to collect and analyze information effectively allows preppers to remain calm, make smart decisions, and protect themselves and their families. By using a combination of traditional and digital sources, cross-referencing details, and practicing patience, preppers can stay aware and responsive, no matter how challenging the crisis. Information can often be the deciding factor between chaos and safety, making it one of the most important tools for anyone dedicated to preparedness.

CHAPTER 6

Transportation and Evacuation

Preparing Reliable Transportation for Emergencies

In emergencies, having reliable transportation can mean the difference between staying safe and being stranded. Whether it's evacuating due to a natural disaster or needing to reach a secure location, being prepared with a dependable vehicle is essential. Reliable transportation not only helps you reach a safe destination, but it also gives you the flexibility to transport supplies, navigate difficult terrains, and even help others if necessary. Preparing a vehicle with the right gear and maintaining it properly is an important part of emergency planning.

The first step in vehicle preparedness is ensuring that your car is in good working condition at all times. Regular maintenance, such as oil changes, brake inspections, and tire rotations, helps prevent mechanical failures during critical moments. Checking the vehicle's battery, lights, and wiper blades also ensures that it can function reliably, even in rough weather or low visibility. Having a trusted mechanic inspect your vehicle periodically adds an extra layer of reassurance that your car is ready when you need it most.

Keeping a sufficient fuel supply is another crucial part of transportation readiness. In a crisis, gas stations can quickly run out of fuel, or power outages may make pumps inoperable. It's a good habit to keep your fuel tank at least half full at all times, as this minimizes the chance of running out unexpectedly. Additionally, storing a few extra gallons of fuel in a safe, approved container can serve as a backup. If you rely on gasoline storage, remember to keep it in a well-ventilated, cool area away from direct sunlight, as it is highly flammable.

Besides fuel, it's essential to equip your vehicle with emergency supplies. Basic items, such as a first-aid kit, flashlight, water, non-perishable food, and blankets, should be stored in the car. These items can be life-saving if you end up stranded or facing unexpected delays. For instance, bottled water can prevent dehydration on long drives, and blankets help keep you warm in cold weather if you need to stop for extended periods. Adding high-energy snacks like protein bars or trail mix also provides a reliable source of nourishment.

In addition to essentials, some extra tools and equipment are highly useful in emergencies. A quality spare tire, jack, and tire iron allow you to change a flat if needed. Jumper cables or a portable battery pack can help if your vehicle's battery dies unexpectedly. Having a fire extinguisher on hand can also address small fires that may occur in the vehicle. A multi-tool, which includes pliers, screwdrivers, and a knife, is versatile and can be helpful for repairs or emergencies. Keep these items stored securely in your vehicle to avoid clutter and ensure they're easily accessible.

For those who live in areas prone to extreme weather or rough terrain, having a vehicle with off-road capability may be beneficial. Off-road vehicles, such as SUVs or trucks with four-wheel drive, are generally better equipped to handle muddy, rocky, or flooded roads. If flooding or landslides occur, such a vehicle is more likely to navigate these conditions safely. Even if your primary vehicle isn't off-road capable, ensuring it has solid traction and good quality tires helps improve its performance on rougher roads.

Navigation is another essential aspect of vehicle readiness. Although GPS devices and smartphones are extremely useful, they can fail in remote areas or when cell networks are down. Having a physical map of your region or a reliable GPS unit that doesn't depend on cell service can be valuable in emergencies. Mark potential evacuation routes, safe locations, and places where you could potentially stop for supplies or fuel. Familiarize yourself with these routes before an emergency arises so you're not figuring it out under pressure.

If an evacuation order is issued, being able to load essential supplies into the vehicle quickly can save valuable time. It's helpful to have a basic "go-bag" or emergency kit stored in your car, containing personal identification, important documents, medications, phone chargers, and cash. Additionally, consider organizing supplies in storage containers or bags that can be easily carried. Keeping items organized minimizes the chance of forgetting something important in a rush and allows you to make the best use of your vehicle's space.

Another important consideration is how to pack your vehicle effectively for maximum efficiency and accessibility. Place heavier items, like water and canned goods, on the floor or lower areas to keep the vehicle stable. Secure loose items so they don't move around while driving. Items that you may need to access quickly, like the first-aid kit, flashlight, or snacks, should be stored in an easy-to-reach location, such as the glove compartment or a seat organizer. Organizing supplies carefully makes the vehicle not only more comfortable but also safer for all passengers.

In emergency situations, the ability to communicate and stay informed is vital. Keep a portable phone charger or a power bank in the car, so you can recharge your phone even if the vehicle's battery dies. A two-way radio or CB radio can be useful in situations where cell networks are down, as they enable you to receive updates from others nearby. If you frequently travel in rural or isolated areas, consider a satellite phone for long-range communication, as it works independently of cell towers.

Preparing mentally for emergency transportation is just as important as the physical preparation of your vehicle. Practice safe driving habits at all times, including obeying speed limits, wearing seatbelts, and staying aware of road conditions. If you're faced with an evacuation, stay calm and avoid taking unnecessary risks, such as speeding or ignoring traffic signs. When traveling through congested or unfamiliar routes, patience and alertness will help you make better decisions and keep yourself and others safe.

Understanding and practicing alternative transportation methods may also come in handy if your vehicle becomes unusable. Bicycles, for example, are easy to maintain and don't require fuel, making them a reliable alternative for short distances. In more rural or remote locations, ATVs or utility vehicles may be suitable alternatives for transportation through tough terrain. Thinking about these options in advance can prepare you for scenarios where traditional vehicles may not be the best choice.

In any emergency, knowing how to safely evacuate by vehicle requires not only the right equipment but also a clear plan. Planning several routes to safe locations; taking into account possible road closures, traffic jams, and hazards is critical. Share these routes and your plan with family or friends so they know where to expect you. If you're part of a larger group or have family members to consider, ensure everyone knows their roles and understands the evacuation plan, making the process smoother and faster.

To keep your vehicle emergency-ready over the long term, establish a regular routine for checking supplies and equipment. Periodically inspect stored items like water, food, and batteries to ensure they haven't expired or been used. Replace any items that are past their best-use date, and restock supplies as needed. Additionally, check your fuel supply regularly and refresh any stored gasoline to keep it from going stale.

Having a reliable mode of transportation during emergencies is crucial for safety and survival. By maintaining your vehicle, stocking it with emergency supplies, and being prepared for various scenarios, you ensure that you can respond quickly and effectively in a crisis. The right preparation helps not only in protecting yourself but also in supporting others, whether through evacuation, supply transportation, or communication. With a dependable vehicle and a well-prepared plan, you're far more equipped to face any emergency with confidence and resilience.

Evacuation Plans and Vehicle Prep for Safe Exit

Creating a solid evacuation plan is essential for responding safely to emergency situations. Whether it's a natural disaster, unexpected evacuation order, or any crisis that requires leaving quickly, having a well-thought-out plan can help reduce stress and ensure everyone's safety. An evacuation plan includes multiple escape routes, chosen safe destinations, and a vehicle that's prepared for quick departure. By planning ahead, you can be ready to evacuate swiftly, safely, and with the supplies you need.

The first step in an evacuation plan is to identify safe destinations where you can take shelter. These could include the homes of trusted friends or family members, community shelters, or designated emergency locations. Ideally, choose destinations in different directions to provide options depending on the nature of the emergency. For instance, if a storm is moving from the north, having an evacuation spot to the south is useful. Check if the chosen destination has amenities like electricity, water, and communication capabilities. Knowing in advance where you will go can provide peace of mind and help everyone involved stay calm and focused during the evacuation.

It's also important to have multiple evacuation routes planned in case roads are blocked, heavily congested, or unsafe. Start by looking at a detailed map of your area, marking the primary route to each safe destination. Then, identify at least two alternative routes for each destination. Take note of any major landmarks, intersections, or highways that could serve as key points on these routes. Try to avoid routes that rely on a single road or bridge, as these can become bottlenecks during mass evacuations. Practice driving these routes when possible so that you and any family members know them well.

When planning routes, consider possible road conditions. For instance, floods or landslides can make certain roads impassable. If your area is prone to heavy traffic, such as during rush hours, try to plan routes that avoid major intersections or busy highways. Additionally, if any part of your evacuation plan involves backroads, ensure these routes are safe for your vehicle type, especially if they involve unpaved or rough terrain. Taking these factors into account while mapping out routes helps you avoid delays and minimize risk when it's time to evacuate.

Vehicle readiness is equally critical in an evacuation plan. A well-maintained vehicle with adequate fuel is essential for a safe, smooth evacuation. Regularly check oil levels, brakes, tires, and other essential components of your vehicle. Also, ensure the tank is kept at least half full at all times to avoid stopping at gas stations when fuel may be in short supply. Additionally, if possible, store extra fuel in approved containers, but always handle it with care and store it safely outside of the vehicle's main cabin to reduce risks.

Having the right type of vehicle can also make a big difference in an evacuation. Vehicles with off-road capabilities, such as SUVs, trucks, or other four-wheel-drive models, are often ideal for emergencies. These vehicles can handle unpaved roads, minor obstacles, or areas with poor road conditions. While smaller, fuel-efficient cars are also useful for covering long distances without frequent fuel stops, their performance may be limited on rough terrain. If you live in an area where off-road travel could be necessary, a vehicle equipped with four-wheel drive and solid traction is a strong choice for added security and versatility.

Packing your vehicle effectively can improve the speed and safety of your evacuation. Essential supplies, such as water, non-perishable food, first-aid kits, and blankets, should be stored in easy-to-access areas within the car. Additionally, bring any critical documents, including IDs, insurance papers, and emergency contact lists. Secure these items in a waterproof folder or bag to protect them from damage. If possible, divide items into clear categories and store them in separate containers. This organization helps reduce clutter and allows you to find things quickly when needed.

It's helpful to have emergency tools and equipment on hand in your vehicle, as they can be essential if you encounter unexpected challenges. For instance, a high-quality spare tire, jack, and tire iron are necessary for fixing flat tires. Jumper cables or a portable battery pack can be invaluable if the battery dies. Additionally, a fire extinguisher, flashlight, and multi-tool can assist with a range of small repairs or issues that might arise along the way. Keeping these tools within reach is key to a successful and safe journey during an evacuation.

Communication plays a vital role in any evacuation plan. Have a fully charged phone, portable charger, and car charger in the vehicle to ensure your phone stays powered. If cellular networks are down, consider using two-way radios or CB radios to stay connected with others. In case you have to inform loved ones of your location, having a way to communicate can reduce worry and help coordinate efforts. Additionally, make sure everyone involved in the evacuation plan knows where you're headed and the routes you're planning to take.

For large families or groups, coordinate everyone's roles before an emergency occurs. This means designating one person to navigate, another to keep track of supplies, and others to assist in loading the vehicle if necessary. Make sure each person knows what they need to do, especially children, who may feel less scared if they understand the plan and have a simple responsibility, like carrying their own go-bag. Practicing the evacuation plan as a family or group makes it feel more natural and reduces confusion when it's time to act.

Preparation doesn't end with packing your vehicle; practice loading supplies and driving along designated routes periodically. This practice helps everyone know what to expect and how to react in real-time. Being familiar with the packing process speeds up the departure and reduces the risk of leaving behind critical items. Regular drills are an effective way to identify any issues with your plan, such as adjusting supply placement, refining routes, or recognizing if additional items are needed.

Pets and animals should also be considered in your evacuation plan. Have a pet carrier or secure crate ready, along with supplies such as food, water, and any medications your pets may need. Make sure the vehicle has enough space for pets to travel comfortably, as frightened animals can become unpredictable. Identifying pet-friendly shelters in advance can be very helpful, especially if you need to stay at one of your chosen safe destinations for an extended period.

An emergency kit or go-bag that stays in the vehicle at all times can add to your readiness. Include basic items like water, snacks, a flashlight, first-aid supplies, and any necessary medications. This bag should be periodically checked and refreshed to ensure all items are current and functional. By keeping this bag in the car, you add an extra layer of security, ensuring you have essentials even if you need to leave in a hurry.

Creating a comprehensive evacuation plan that includes multiple routes, reliable destinations, and a well-prepared vehicle can help you navigate emergencies with confidence. Regularly review your routes, update supplies, and make sure everyone involved understands their role. By carefully planning and practicing, you equip yourself and those around you with the knowledge and resources to evacuate safely and efficiently, no matter the emergency.

Alternative Travel Options for Survival

In situations where traditional vehicles like cars or trucks are unavailable or impractical, having alternative transportation options is key to survival. Whether due to fuel shortages, road blockages, or the need for stealth, being able to rely on methods like bicycles, motorcycles, or even walking can make all the difference in reaching safety. Preparing for these options requires careful planning, the right equipment, and knowledge of how to optimize each method for efficient travel, especially under challenging conditions.

Bicycles are one of the best alternative transportation methods in emergency situations. They're quiet, don't require fuel, and can navigate narrow trails, sidewalks, or even forest paths that are inaccessible to larger vehicles. When choosing a bicycle for survival purposes, it's best to go with a sturdy, all-terrain or mountain bike, as these are built to handle rougher surfaces. Ensure the bike has a reliable braking system, thick tires, and a comfortable seat. If possible, add a front or rear rack to carry supplies and use waterproof bags or panniers to protect items from the elements.

Regular maintenance is crucial for any bike you plan to use in emergencies. Check the tires, chain, and gears frequently, making sure they're in good condition. Carry a basic bike repair kit that includes a tire pump, patch kit, extra inner tubes, and a multi-tool to handle repairs on the go. Practice riding with a loaded bike to get a sense of how it feels and understand any limitations. Bicycles also allow you to travel faster than walking while expending less energy, which is valuable when covering long distances.

Motorcycles offer a faster alternative than bicycles, especially over long distances or open areas, but they do come with some challenges. A motorcycle needs fuel, so in emergency situations, it's wise to carry a portable fuel container if possible. Choose a reliable, off-road motorcycle or dual-sport bike that can handle uneven terrain, and make sure it's equipped with strong tires that provide traction. Motorcycles are compact enough to maneuver around obstacles, making them ideal for escaping through traffic jams or traveling along narrow trails.

Safety gear like a helmet, gloves, and sturdy boots are necessary when using a motorcycle. It's also a good idea to carry tools for basic maintenance, including extra spark plugs, a wrench set, and spare parts for common repairs. Practice handling the bike on rougher terrain if you expect to travel off-road, as this type of riding can be very different from navigating paved streets. Motorcycles are efficient for solo travel or carrying one passenger, but their limited cargo space means you'll need to pack only the essentials.

Walking may be the most accessible, yet slowest, form of travel during an emergency. While it lacks the speed of bicycles and motorcycles, walking has the advantage of flexibility. You can navigate through virtually any terrain, including thick forests, mountains, or urban areas, and it requires no fuel or maintenance. To prepare for walking long distances, choose durable, weather-resistant clothing, and invest in high-quality hiking boots that offer both comfort and support. Blisters, sore muscles, and fatigue are common issues, so it's important to build up your endurance beforehand.

When walking, carry only the most essential items to avoid being weighed down. A sturdy backpack is crucial, with padded shoulder straps and a waist belt to distribute the weight. Organize supplies so that frequently needed items, like water, snacks, and navigation tools, are easily accessible. Consider packing items like a portable water filter, rain gear, and a lightweight sleeping bag in case you need to rest outdoors. Having a map and compass can help you navigate if electronic devices lose power, and a reliable flashlight will allow you to keep moving even at night.

For longer trips on foot, think about pacing yourself and taking breaks to avoid exhaustion. Plan a route that includes sources of water, shade, and safe places to rest if possible. It's also helpful to have a mental list of landmarks along the way, as these can guide you and provide reassurance. Preparing physically by walking and hiking regularly before an emergency can build stamina and help you feel more comfortable carrying a backpack.

Other forms of alternative transportation may be less common but still useful in certain scenarios. Boats or kayaks, for example, can be valuable if you live near water and need to evacuate quickly. Inflatable rafts are compact and can be stored in your car or home, allowing you to cross bodies of water if necessary. Like with bicycles and motorcycles, make sure you're familiar with using and maintaining these watercraft and carry any needed gear, such as paddles, life vests, and waterproof storage for essentials.

Horses and other animals are another potential option in rural areas or places where modern transportation is limited. While horses need food, water, and rest, they can carry both people and supplies over long distances and rough terrain. If you have access to horses, be sure they're trained for trail riding and able to carry loaded saddlebags. Learning basic care, including feeding, grooming, and handling, will ensure your horse is healthy and prepared for an emergency.

Preparing for alternative transportation also means considering the supplies you'll need. Survival essentials like water, food, first-aid kits, and navigation tools should always be packed, regardless of your travel method. Lightweight gear is key to minimizing strain, especially for bicycles, motorcycles, and walking. Dehydrated meals, compact water filters, and solar-powered chargers are all smart choices, allowing you to stay prepared without weighing yourself down.

Communication devices are equally important. A portable two-way radio, satellite phone, or personal locator beacon can help you call for assistance if needed. While mobile phones are convenient, they may not work in remote areas or during disasters that disrupt networks. Practice using any communication devices beforehand so you understand how they function and how to get help.

Preparing for different transportation methods also involves planning routes that are suitable for each mode. While a motorcycle may work well on a major road, bicycles and walking routes might take you through quieter paths, forest trails, or even alleyways. Always assess the safety of a route before traveling, considering factors like visibility, possible hazards, and access to resources.

Training and practice are essential for each type of transportation. Familiarity with handling and repairing bikes, motorcycles, or boats can boost your confidence and efficiency. Likewise, practicing hiking with a loaded backpack can prepare you for the challenges of walking over long distances. By becoming comfortable with each method, you're better prepared to make quick decisions and stay safe in unpredictable situations.

By having multiple transportation options and knowing how to prepare for each, you increase your chances of successfully reaching a safe destination. Flexibility and adaptability are key when vehicles are unavailable, allowing you to respond to changing conditions with resilience. The time invested in preparation, physical training, and equipment maintenance will ensure you're ready for any journey, whether it's by bicycle, motorcycle, or on foot.

CHAPTER 7

Financial Preparedness

Building Financial Resilience in Anticipation of Crisis

Financial resilience is a critical part of preparedness, giving you a strong foundation to handle emergencies without overwhelming stress. Financial preparedness means having the ability to weather unexpected situations, whether they're natural disasters, economic downturns, or even personal crises. Having a strategy in place to save, invest, and secure assets helps reduce vulnerability and ensures stability. Building financial resilience requires a mix of saving, smart investing, debt management, and understanding how to protect assets from risks. By creating a financial safety net, you increase your capacity to manage challenging times with greater peace of mind.

A first step in building financial resilience is to develop a consistent savings habit. Setting aside a portion of your income each month may seem small, but over time, it grows into a reliable fund. Start by building an emergency fund that can cover at least three to six months of essential expenses, such as housing, food, and utilities. This fund acts as a financial cushion, allowing you to manage unexpected expenses without relying on credit or loans. Keeping the fund in a savings account that's easily accessible ensures you can use it when needed without penalties or delays.

Beyond basic savings, consider diversifying your investments. Having a mix of assets, such as stocks, bonds, real estate, and precious metals, reduces the impact of market changes on your finances. Diversification works by spreading your investments across various sectors, so if one area suffers a loss, others may remain stable or even grow. For example, during economic downturns, stocks may lose value, but precious metals like gold and silver often retain or increase in worth. Holding a small amount of physical gold or silver can provide a backup source of value that's easy to store and transport.

Another way to secure assets is to invest in real estate, which offers both a place to live and an asset that generally appreciates over time. If purchasing property isn't an option, investing in Real Estate Investment Trusts allows you to benefit from real estate investments with less upfront cost. Real Estate Investment Trusts provide dividends, which can serve as an additional income stream. They're also more liquid than physical property, meaning you can sell shares if you need cash. Diversifying your assets helps you avoid putting all your resources into a single area, which protects you against unexpected market swings.

In addition to investing, consider securing your finances by reducing debt. Debt, especially high-interest debt, can drain your resources during emergencies. Focus on paying off credit card balances, personal loans, and other high-interest debts first. By eliminating or reducing these debts, you free up funds for more important expenses and reduce the risk of falling into a cycle of debt. Budgeting can help you track spending, prioritize debt payments, and identify areas where you can save. Once high-interest debts are managed, you can focus on building wealth instead of managing monthly payments.

Another aspect of financial preparedness is asset protection. For example, insurance can provide significant protection in a crisis. Health insurance, property insurance, and even disability insurance help safeguard against unforeseen medical costs, damage to assets, or loss of income. Regularly reviewing insurance policies ensures you're adequately covered and that any changes in your life or assets are reflected in your protection plans. In addition, setting up a will or a trust provides clear instructions for how your assets should be handled, offering peace of mind for you and security for your loved ones.

Diversifying your income streams can also reduce financial vulnerability. Relying solely on one job or source of income can be risky if that source is disrupted. Explore side businesses, freelance work, or passive income options, such as rental income, dividends, or royalties. Having multiple income streams means you're less likely to face a complete loss of income if one source is affected. Even a small side income can make a big difference in strengthening your financial safety net.

Another key to financial resilience is having a well-thought-out financial plan. This plan includes setting clear goals, such as how much you want to save, how much debt to eliminate, and which assets to invest in. Review and adjust your plan regularly to keep up with life changes, such as a new job, a move, or a significant expense. Tracking your financial progress motivates you to stay on course, and adjustments can be made as your priorities evolve. A flexible financial plan adapts to change, allowing you to navigate unexpected events with greater confidence.

It's also wise to have a small amount of cash on hand for emergencies, especially for situations where digital payment systems are unavailable. Cash ensures you can still buy essentials, like food and gas, even if banks or credit card networks are down. Store this cash in a safe place, and make sure it's accessible if you need it in a hurry. Alongside cash, prepaid cards or secure digital wallets with some funds can offer extra options for emergencies, making you less dependent on traditional banking.

In addition to preparing financially, it's essential to educate yourself on financial literacy. Understanding the basics of budgeting, investing, and risk management gives you greater control over your resources. Learning about economic trends, inflation, and potential risks to your finances allows you to make informed decisions. For example, knowing how inflation affects purchasing power can guide you in choosing the best places to store your savings. By building financial knowledge, you make it easier to adapt your strategy to changing conditions.

Community support is also a valuable part of financial resilience. Having a network of family, friends, or local community members with whom you can share resources or skills reduces strain during tough times. For example, swapping skills like gardening or repairs saves money on outsourced services. If financial collapse occurs, having a reliable support system can offer mutual assistance, increasing everyone's chances of coping well. Additionally, community resources, such as food banks or local credit unions, often provide aid during emergencies, helping individuals and families manage immediate needs.

Practicing mindful spending habits contributes to financial resilience, too. By focusing on needs over wants, you can save more and avoid impulse purchases that might strain your budget. Minimalism, or the practice of simplifying possessions and spending only on essentials, helps maintain financial stability. Developing these habits also builds self-discipline, making it easier to stick to your financial plan and prioritize savings.

Keeping an eye on potential risks and future trends also strengthens financial preparedness. Monitoring news about economic indicators, natural disasters, or political developments helps you stay aware of factors that might impact your finances. For instance, if inflation rates are rising, adjusting your budget and focusing on preserving purchasing power might be necessary. Keeping informed about potential financial or environmental changes allows you to make proactive decisions and reduce your risk of financial loss.

Remember that financial preparedness is an ongoing process. Building resilience takes time and requires steady effort, but it pays off by providing stability and reducing stress during emergencies. Staying consistent in your financial habits, updating your strategies, and maintaining flexibility helps you stay prepared no matter what life brings. By focusing on long-term financial resilience, you're creating a more secure foundation that can support you and your loved ones in any crisis.

Money Management Strategies for Preppers

Managing money effectively is essential during any emergency, helping to make sure resources last as long as possible. In a crisis, you might have limited access to your regular income, making it crucial to have a clear financial plan that focuses on budgeting, cutting unnecessary expenses, and finding alternative ways to access essentials through cash and barter systems. Having financial flexibility is also important because it allows you to adapt quickly to changing conditions and unexpected expenses. The following strategies are designed to help you stretch your resources, maintain stability, and stay prepared for any situation that arises.

One of the most effective money management strategies during a crisis is setting up a realistic and carefully considered budget. A crisis budget should focus only on essential expenses, such as food, water, shelter, and any necessary medical supplies. Start by listing your available funds and estimating how long you'll need to make them last. This budget might look different from your usual monthly budget, as it focuses solely on immediate survival needs. Avoid spending on non-essential items, and make adjustments as the situation changes. Tracking every purchase, no matter how small, keeps you accountable and helps you see exactly where your money is going.

Alongside budgeting, reducing unnecessary expenses is critical. During an emergency, some costs that may have been a part of your regular budget may no longer be necessary or practical. For example, subscription services, dining out, or entertainment expenses are likely to become low priorities. Cutting back on these costs frees up more money for essentials. Reassess your recurring bills and consider temporarily canceling anything that isn't strictly necessary. For recurring utility or service costs, consider negotiating for lower rates if possible. Many service providers may offer temporary assistance programs during crises.

Cash is a valuable resource during emergencies, especially if banking systems or electronic payments are disrupted. Having cash on hand ensures you can still buy essential items if digital systems go down. Small bills are particularly useful, as they make it easier to pay for items without needing change. Storing a set amount of cash in a secure but easily accessible place is recommended. Keep this emergency cash in a waterproof and fireproof container, ensuring that it's ready if you need it. While cash is ideal for immediate purchases, be mindful to only use it when absolutely necessary, as it may be hard to replenish.

In addition to cash, the barter system can be a practical method for obtaining goods and services in situations where money may not be useful. Bartering is the exchange of goods or services without using money, allowing you to trade items you have for ones you need. For instance, if you have extra food supplies but lack medical items, you might find someone willing to trade. Commonly bartered items include non-perishable food, batteries, medical supplies, and personal care items. Essential skills, like first aid, repairs, or gardening, can also be valuable in a barter situation. To successfully use bartering, take inventory of your supplies and skills, and look for others with complementary resources.

Maintaining financial flexibility is key in managing funds during an emergency. Flexibility means being prepared to adjust your budget, find new sources of income, or make changes to your spending habits as circumstances evolve. Flexibility could include learning how to repair your own items instead of buying new ones or being open to using alternative resources when supplies are low. Being willing to make difficult financial decisions on the spot and adapt to sudden changes ensures that your money lasts as long as possible. Financial flexibility is easier to maintain if you already have a range of practical skills and a diverse set of resources at your disposal.

Using alternative payment methods can also be helpful during an emergency. Prepaid debit cards, for example, are another form of secure payment that can be loaded with a set amount of money. These cards are usually not tied to a bank account, so if you lose access to your regular funds, prepaid cards can serve as a backup. Digital wallets on secure devices might offer another way to store and access funds. However, these options rely on digital infrastructure, so have them only as secondary options to cash and barter. Also, maintain a list of local businesses that accept alternative forms of payment or are known for offering credit during emergencies.

Another important aspect of emergency money management is finding creative ways to increase your funds or resources. If possible, look for temporary work or freelance opportunities that fit within the current situation. Many remote jobs, like writing, design, or customer service, can be done from home if internet access is available. If in-person work is an option, tasks like delivery driving, yard work, or essential trade skills might provide temporary income. Think outside the box by finding ways to leverage any items or skills you have to earn extra money or supplies.

Learning to differentiate between needs and wants also plays a major role in emergency money management. Needs are things you must have to survive, while wants are things you can do without. Prioritizing needs over wants helps you conserve your resources and focus on essentials. Practice asking yourself whether each purchase is truly necessary. This habit can lead to smarter spending decisions, both during a crisis and afterward. Needs may vary slightly depending on your personal or family situation, so tailor your budget and priorities to what's most essential for survival and well-being.

Saving and rationing resources is another practical strategy. If you have a stockpile of food, medicine, or other essentials, ration these supplies to extend their use. Practice controlled consumption, using only what is necessary each day. This habit conserves resources for a longer period and may also allow you to help others in need, should the opportunity arise. Maintaining a stockpile also reduces the amount of money you need to spend on supplies, freeing up funds for any unexpected expenses that arise.

A clear record of expenses and resources can be extremely useful. Keeping a simple log of all purchases and trades, along with an inventory of supplies, allows you to monitor how quickly you're using items and where you may need to restock. This log also helps you notice patterns, like areas where you're spending too much, so you can adjust your budget as needed. Documenting every transaction, whether it's with cash, barter, or alternative payments, ensures you know exactly where your resources stand.

Planning ahead, even in the middle of a crisis, prepares you for potential shifts in circumstances. If you anticipate that certain goods might become scarce, focus on securing them as soon as possible. Recognize that prices may rise during emergencies, so purchasing early when possible may save money in the long run. Anticipate the possibility of increased utility costs if you're relying on power or water more heavily, and adjust your budget accordingly. Thinking a few steps ahead in terms of resource needs and financial spending gives you an advantage in managing finances throughout an extended emergency.

Building a habit of resourcefulness and resilience in money management creates stability, even during uncertain times. Resourcefulness means making the most of what you already have, whether that's by repairing items, repurposing supplies, or finding innovative uses for common objects. This approach saves money by avoiding unnecessary purchases. Resilience, on the other hand, is the ability to handle financial stress without panicking. Cultivating a mindset that can adapt to financial challenges with creativity and a calm approach leads to better decision-making and helps you stay on course through any crisis.

Financial preparedness and effective money management can significantly improve your chances of stability and security during emergencies. Each strategy—from budgeting and expense reduction to cash use, bartering, and financial flexibility—contributes to a stronger foundation in times of crisis. By developing these skills and habits, you'll be better equipped to manage resources wisely, face financial challenges, and remain resilient in the face of uncertainty. This level of financial preparedness ultimately enhances your ability to provide for yourself and your loved ones in any situation.

Barter Systems and Trading for Survival

A barter system is an exchange method where goods and services are traded directly without using money. In times of crisis, when cash may lose its value or become inaccessible, bartering can become a crucial way for people to meet their needs. This system has been used for centuries and often becomes essential during emergencies, as it allows individuals to obtain necessities by exchanging items they already have. Understanding how a barter system works, knowing what makes certain items valuable, and learning negotiation strategies are all essential skills for survival in a barter economy.

Barter systems operate on the principle of mutual benefit: each person involved in a trade provides something the other needs or values. For example, if someone has extra canned food but needs medical supplies, they could find someone with a surplus of medical items who might need food. The trade is then made based on the agreement of both parties. Unlike traditional transactions with set prices, barter deals depend on personal negotiation and the specific needs of each person. As a result, every trade may look different, and the "value" of items can vary depending on the urgency of needs and availability of resources.

In a barter system, items with practical value often become the most sought-after. Essentials like food, water, hygiene products, medical supplies, and clothing hold high trade value because they directly impact survival and well-being. Non-perishable food items, such as canned goods, dried beans, and rice, are particularly useful in bartering because they last a long time and are easy to store. Other valuable items include tools, batteries, and alternative power sources, which can help people maintain a basic level of comfort and safety in challenging conditions. Fuel, cooking supplies, and lighting sources like candles or lanterns also become valuable, as they support basic daily functions when modern conveniences may be limited.

Another category of valuable trade items includes hygiene products and medications. In emergencies, these items can be scarce, and maintaining cleanliness and health is essential to prevent illness. Therefore, personal care items like soap, toothpaste, feminine hygiene products, and disinfectants often have high trade value. Medications, even basic ones like pain relievers, antibiotics, and allergy medicine, are in demand since they directly impact health. If you have a supply of these essentials, they can be excellent items to trade with others who need them.

Skills can also be valuable in a barter economy. If you're skilled in first aid, repair work, or gardening, these abilities can serve as barter assets. Instead of trading physical items, you might offer a service in exchange for goods. For example, someone with medical knowledge could offer treatment in exchange for food or supplies. Those skilled in repair work could fix tools or build shelter in exchange for other essentials. Having valuable skills gives you an edge in a barter economy, as you're able to provide something that might not be as easily obtainable as physical items.

When approaching bartering, negotiation skills become essential. Since there are no fixed prices, it's important to know how to assess the value of what you have and what you need. Start by being clear about your priorities; know what you need the most and what items or skills you can afford to trade. When negotiating, it's often helpful to begin with an offer that leaves room for adjustments. This way, you can make concessions if necessary, without sacrificing too much value. It's also wise to have a few alternatives ready in case the person you're trading with has different needs. Flexibility can make negotiations smoother, allowing both parties to find common ground more easily.

Understanding the value of items in relation to scarcity is another key aspect of bartering effectively. In a crisis, certain items may be extremely hard to come by, which increases their value significantly. For instance, clean water or purification tablets may be priceless in a situation where water is scarce. Similarly, fuel becomes highly valuable when electricity is unavailable. Keeping track of which resources are limited and high in demand gives you an advantage, as it allows you to anticipate which items will be most valuable in trades. Conversely, items that are widely available may have less trade value, so be mindful of the market conditions within the barter system.

Building trust with the people you barter with can also make future exchanges easier. Trustworthy trading partners are more likely to make fair deals and may prioritize trades with you in the future. Honesty and transparency help build this trust—communicate clearly about the condition of the items you're trading and be reliable in honoring any agreements made. Additionally, developing a network of trusted barter partners provides you with more options, allowing you to find better deals and access a wider range of resources. Establishing good relationships can benefit both parties and create a sense of mutual support in challenging times.

Preparation is another important aspect of bartering effectively. Before entering a barter system, consider which items you may be able to trade and start setting aside extras. If possible, create a small stockpile of high-value items, specifically those that are easy to store and have long shelf lives. Even small quantities of certain items, like batteries or painkillers, can become valuable in a trade. Having a prepared selection of trade items increases your options and gives you more leverage during negotiations. Additionally, keep items organized and in good condition, as the quality of goods also affects their trade value.

In a barter system, being mindful of safety is crucial. As people in need may become more desperate, there is a potential risk of theft or violence. Conduct trades in safe locations, preferably in areas where you're not isolated. If possible, avoid revealing the full extent of your resources to others, as this can make you a target. Storing trade items separately from your main supplies can also help maintain privacy and security. Establishing basic safety protocols helps protect both your resources and your personal well-being while engaging in the barter system.

Remember that bartering is not just about survival but also about community. In a crisis, people often depend on each other for mutual support, and bartering provides a way to strengthen these connections. Treating each trade as an opportunity to build relationships helps foster cooperation, which benefits everyone involved. By focusing on fair and respectful exchanges, you can create a more positive environment, one where people feel supported and connected even during difficult times.

Barter systems can be vital in a crisis, offering a flexible and effective way to exchange goods and services. Knowing the types of items and skills that hold high trade value, practicing negotiation skills, and being prepared with valuable items all contribute to successful bartering. Additionally, focusing on trust, safety, and community relationships adds stability to the barter economy, ensuring that trades remain fair and beneficial. Embracing these strategies makes it easier to adapt to a barter-based system, helping you stay resilient and resourceful no matter the situation.

CHAPTER 8

Health and Wellness

Staying Physically and Mentally Strong in Emergencies

Maintaining physical and mental strength during emergencies is essential for survival and well-being. Challenging times can impact our health in many ways, so it's crucial to focus on keeping our bodies and minds in top condition. When situations become unpredictable or stressful, being physically prepared and mentally resilient makes it easier to handle tough moments, make smart decisions, and protect those around us.

Physical health is our first line of defense against any crisis. Keeping our bodies strong, energized, and healthy allows us to react quickly and avoid illness. Exercise plays an important role here.

Regular movement not only strengthens our muscles but also boosts our immune system, making us less susceptible to sickness. Activities that don't require much space or equipment, like stretching, push-ups, and squats, are excellent for keeping active when you may not have access to your usual routines. Walking or jogging, if safe, can also relieve tension and maintain cardiovascular health. By incorporating even small amounts of movement daily, we build endurance and flexibility, which can be critical in stressful situations.

Nutrition is another key aspect of physical health. Eating a balanced diet fuels our bodies and keeps our energy levels steady. In emergencies, our diet might look different, but it's still important to include a variety of foods when possible. Proteins, like beans, nuts, or canned meat, are essential for muscle repair and immune function. Carbohydrates, such as rice, pasta, or oatmeal, provide quick energy, while healthy fats like nuts or oils can keep us fuller for longer. Vitamins and minerals found in canned or dried vegetables and fruits also contribute to immune health. Even if resources are limited, being mindful of eating a mix of nutrients whenever possible helps us stay strong. Planning a stock of non-perishable, nutritious foods can ensure we have enough energy to get through challenging times.

Hygiene is often overlooked in emergencies but is vital for preventing disease. Washing hands regularly and keeping cooking and eating areas clean can reduce the risk of infections. When water is limited, consider using sanitizers or wipes to clean hands and surfaces. Proper waste management, such as disposing of trash and maintaining clean toilet areas, also minimizes exposure to bacteria. By staying clean, we create a safer environment and reduce the chances of sickness, which is especially important when medical help might be harder to access.

Mental health is just as important as physical health in emergencies. Stress and fear are natural responses to difficult situations, but managing these emotions is crucial for clear thinking. Taking deep breaths or practicing mindfulness can help calm the mind. Mindfulness involves focusing on the present moment and slowing down our thoughts. Even a few minutes of quiet time each day, such as listening to calming sounds or breathing deeply, can help reduce stress. This allows us to make thoughtful decisions, rather than acting on panic or impulse, which can lead to mistakes. Keeping a notebook for writing down thoughts or feelings can also be helpful for mental clarity and emotional relief.

Physical activity also has benefits for mental health. Exercise releases endorphins, chemicals that naturally improve mood and relieve stress. Moving around, even with basic stretches, can make us feel more grounded and positive. Staying active also helps release tension, which is essential when situations feel intense or overwhelming. These little boosts to our mental health help us face challenges more confidently and feel more capable of handling whatever comes our way.

Sleep is another vital component of mental and physical health. Although sleep might feel difficult to maintain in emergencies, rest is crucial for a clear mind and strong body. Sleep restores our energy and sharpens our focus, allowing us to think more clearly. Establishing a routine, like going to bed at the same time each night, can make a big difference. Creating a quiet, dark, and comfortable space can help, even if resources are limited. If sleep is interrupted or difficult, short naps can still offer recovery and help us function better.

Staying socially connected can also support mental health. Even if we're physically separated from family and friends, staying in touch through phone calls or messages provides comfort and emotional support. Talking to others about fears or challenges often makes them feel more manageable. If it's safe to be with others in person, activities like preparing meals together or sharing tasks can create a sense of community and reduce feelings of loneliness. Teamwork and shared responsibility make survival efforts easier and can boost everyone's spirits.

Practicing optimism, or focusing on positive thoughts, can help maintain mental strength during hard times. Optimism doesn't mean ignoring difficulties, but it does mean finding moments of hope or progress, even if they're small. Reminding ourselves of what's going well or things we're grateful for can bring a sense of peace and balance. This positive outlook keeps morale high, giving us the mental energy to keep going even when things seem tough. Staying focused on solutions and progress encourages resilience and helps us see that challenges are temporary and can be overcome.

In emergencies, maintaining routines as much as possible also supports mental well-being. Having a daily structure, like eating meals at regular times, setting goals for each day, or sticking to personal hygiene habits, creates a sense of normalcy and control. Routines keep us grounded and provide a framework to focus on. This sense of order in our day, even if it's simple, can provide comfort and make us feel more in control of our lives during uncertain times.

Preparing a personal wellness kit that includes essentials for both physical and mental health can be incredibly helpful. Items like vitamins, basic medications, hygiene supplies, and even something comforting like a book or puzzle can go a long way. By having access to small comforts, we give ourselves the tools to handle stress, boredom, and anxiety more effectively. Including items that help us relax, such as a favorite music playlist or a few comforting photos, can also provide relief and bring calm in overwhelming moments.

Physical and mental well-being are intertwined, especially during emergencies. By focusing on both areas, we give ourselves the best chance of staying resilient and capable. Balancing exercise, nutrition, and hygiene with activities that support mental clarity and stress relief strengthens our ability to face whatever comes. Taking these steps to care for our whole self prepares us to navigate tough times with confidence and clarity, ensuring that we can be there for ourselves and others no matter the situation.

Health Maintenance Tips for Long-Term Survival

Maintaining health over the long term is essential for survival, especially when professional medical help might not be available. Staying healthy during challenging times requires a combination of disease prevention, good hygiene practices, regular self-care routines, and basic first aid knowledge. By focusing on these areas, you can keep your body strong and prepared to handle various situations, reducing the risk of sickness and injury while improving your chances of thriving.

Disease prevention starts with keeping yourself and your environment clean. Many diseases spread through germs that live on our hands, shared surfaces, and food. Washing hands often with soap and clean water is one of the best ways to prevent these germs from entering the body. When clean water is limited, hand sanitizers can be helpful, but soap and water are always preferred. Regularly disinfecting surfaces that are touched often, such as doorknobs, counters, and cooking areas, also reduces the spread of harmful bacteria and viruses. A clean environment can prevent a lot of common illnesses from affecting you and those around you.

Water sanitation is equally important. Drinking contaminated water can lead to serious diseases, such as cholera or dysentery, which can be life-threatening if untreated. Boiling water for at least one minute is a simple and effective way to kill bacteria and other harmful organisms. If boiling isn't an option, water purification tablets or filtration systems can make water safer to drink.

Always avoid drinking water from unknown sources without treating it first, and store clean water in closed containers to keep it safe from contamination.

Food safety practices can also prevent illness. Storing food properly, especially perishable items, keeps bacteria from growing and spoiling it. If refrigeration isn't available, dried, canned, or dehydrated foods are better options because they last longer. Raw foods, especially meat, should be cooked thoroughly to kill any harmful organisms. Preparing and handling food with clean hands and using sanitized utensils and surfaces further ensures that bacteria don't get into your meals. Eating safe and clean food is essential for maintaining energy and avoiding health issues that can make survival more challenging.

In addition to hygiene, taking care of your body through self-care routines is crucial. Getting enough rest and sleep allows your body to repair itself and boosts your immune system, making it easier to fight off illnesses. When sleep might be interrupted or limited, even short naps can provide the rest your body needs. Regular physical activity, such as stretching or simple exercises, keeps your muscles and joints flexible and strengthens your heart and lungs. Staying active also improves mental health by reducing stress, which is important when dealing with long-term survival challenges.

Dealing with injuries effectively can prevent them from worsening or leading to infections. For minor cuts or scrapes, cleaning the wound with clean water and applying a bandage is usually enough. For deeper cuts, disinfecting with antiseptic solutions and using sterile bandages can help avoid infection. Keeping a basic first aid kit on hand with supplies like bandages, gauze, tweezers, antiseptic wipes, and pain relievers can be incredibly helpful. Changing bandages daily and keeping wounds clean is important to prevent infection, which can be especially dangerous if medical help is not readily available.

Burns are another common injury that can occur, especially if cooking or heating sources are involved. For minor burns, cool the affected area with running water for several minutes and then cover it with a clean, non-stick bandage. Avoid using ice directly on burns, as it can damage the skin. Aloe vera gel, if available, can be soothing and help with the healing process. For more serious burns, keeping the area clean and covering it loosely until you can access medical help is essential. Burns can lead to infections if not treated properly, so cleanliness and careful monitoring are key.

Infections can become life-threatening without proper care, making prevention and early treatment important. Signs of infection include redness, swelling, warmth, pain, or pus at the site of an injury. If you notice any of these signs, cleaning the wound and applying an antiseptic can help prevent it from spreading. If you have access to antibiotics and know the correct dosage, they can be used as a last resort for serious infections, but it's important to use them responsibly and only when absolutely necessary.

Dealing with illnesses in the absence of professional medical help requires some basic knowledge of symptoms and treatments. Fevers, coughs, sore throats, and digestive issues can all arise and make survival more challenging. Keeping hydrated is one of the best ways to manage fevers, as the body loses water when it's fighting off infections. Warm liquids, honey, and saltwater gargles can help soothe sore throats. For digestive issues, such as diarrhea, staying hydrated with clean water and using oral rehydration salts if available can help prevent dehydration, which can become dangerous over time.

Knowing how to identify and treat dehydration is also important. When the body loses too much water, it affects every part of your health. Signs of dehydration include dry mouth, dark urine, dizziness, and fatigue. Drinking small, frequent sips of water can help if you're feeling dehydrated. In more severe cases, adding a pinch of salt and sugar to water can help restore lost electrolytes. By staying aware of your body's hydration levels and addressing dehydration early, you can avoid further health issues.

Managing chronic health conditions is an important part of long-term health maintenance. If you rely on medication, it's a good idea to keep a supply on hand whenever possible. Proper storage, often in a cool, dry place, helps medications stay effective longer. If professional help isn't available, finding natural remedies or lifestyle changes that can assist with managing conditions might be necessary. For example, people with high blood pressure might reduce salt intake, while those with diabetes may focus on low-sugar foods. Understanding the basics of managing your condition can make a significant difference in maintaining health over the long term.

Mental health care is another key part of staying well. Emergencies and long-term survival can cause stress, anxiety, and feelings of isolation. Taking a few minutes each day to relax, meditate, or engage in calming activities like drawing or writing can help you manage stress. Talking with others if possible can also provide comfort and a sense of normalcy. Keeping a positive outlook, setting small daily goals, and focusing on things you're grateful for can support mental resilience. A healthy mind is crucial for decision-making and emotional strength, especially in challenging circumstances.

Creating a self-care kit with basic supplies can go a long way in keeping you prepared. This might include items like soap, a toothbrush, toothpaste, a washcloth, and any other personal care items that help you stay clean and comfortable. A small mirror can be helpful for self-checking injuries or maintaining hygiene. By having a few essentials available, you can stay clean and feel more in control of your health, even in tough situations.

Long-term survival requires a proactive approach to both physical and mental health. By practicing good hygiene, preventing diseases, staying active, managing injuries, and taking care of your mental well-being, you create a foundation for resilience. With careful attention to these areas, you'll be better prepared to handle the challenges that come with long-term survival, keeping both your body and mind ready to face whatever situations may arise.

Natural Remedies and Alternative Health Practices for Preppers

Natural remedies and alternative health practices are valuable tools for preppers, especially when access to conventional medical care may be limited. Using natural resources like herbs, essential oils, and holistic treatments, preppers can manage minor health issues, support wellness, and prevent certain ailments. These natural methods are easy to learn, often accessible, and can be prepared in advance to ensure you have what you need on hand. By understanding a few key remedies and alternative health practices, you can build a foundation for health and wellness in any situation.

Herbs have been used for centuries as natural treatments for various health issues. They are safe to use when handled properly and offer gentle but effective benefits for common ailments. For instance, ginger is well-known for soothing upset stomachs, reducing nausea, and improving digestion. It can be made into tea by steeping fresh ginger slices in hot water. Chamomile is another versatile herb, widely used for its calming properties. Drinking chamomile tea can help with stress, anxiety, and sleep issues. Peppermint is also helpful for headaches and can improve respiratory health. Growing or stocking up on dried herbs like these makes it easy to prepare natural teas, tinctures, and poultices as needed.

Essential oils are another powerful natural remedy that can provide therapeutic benefits through inhalation or topical use. Lavender essential oil is one of the most popular, known for promoting relaxation and sleep. A few drops on a pillow or added to a diffuser can create a calming atmosphere. Tea tree oil is highly valued for its antibacterial and antifungal properties, making it useful for cuts, insect bites, and minor skin irritations. When using essential oils, it's important to dilute them with a carrier oil like coconut or olive oil to avoid skin irritation. Essential oils are easy to store and carry, making them a great addition to any prepper's health kit.

In addition to herbs and essential oils, there are other natural remedies that can be beneficial for various health issues. Honey, for example, is a natural antibiotic and can soothe sore throats and coughs. It can also be used as a wound dressing to prevent infection, as it creates a barrier and keeps the area moist. Apple cider vinegar is another versatile item; it can aid digestion, relieve skin issues, and even help with sore muscles when added to a warm bath. These simple remedies are accessible and can be prepared easily, providing a wide range of uses for maintaining health.

For pain relief, willow bark is known as "nature's aspirin." The bark contains salicin, which has anti-inflammatory properties and can be chewed or brewed into tea to relieve minor aches and pains. Turmeric is another effective anti-inflammatory, often used for joint pain or arthritis. A mixture of turmeric powder and water can be applied to the skin or consumed in warm milk to reduce inflammation. By having a few pain-relieving herbs and remedies, you can manage discomfort naturally without relying solely on medication.

Managing respiratory issues naturally can be particularly helpful in survival situations. Eucalyptus is excellent for supporting respiratory health. A few drops of eucalyptus oil in hot water can be inhaled as steam to clear congestion and soothe coughs. Thyme, too, has respiratory benefits; it's an expectorant, helping to clear mucus from the lungs. Thyme tea can be made by steeping dried leaves in hot water, and it can help with coughs and colds. Knowing which natural remedies support respiratory health is useful for managing symptoms of colds or seasonal allergies.

Boosting the immune system is important for preventing illness, and there are natural ways to do this. Elderberry is one of the best immune-supporting remedies, especially during cold and flu season. Elderberry syrup or tea is high in antioxidants and can help reduce the duration of illness. Garlic is another immune booster, with antibacterial and antiviral properties. Eating fresh garlic or adding it to meals can help strengthen the body's defenses. Vitamin C-rich foods like oranges, bell peppers, and strawberries also play a vital role in immune health and are easy to incorporate into a diet or store as supplements.

Holistic health practices can also play a crucial role in maintaining well-being. Techniques like meditation and deep breathing exercises help manage stress and promote mental clarity. When facing difficult situations, these practices can reduce anxiety and help you stay focused. Stretching and gentle yoga movements are also helpful for keeping muscles flexible, improving blood circulation, and reducing tension. Practicing mindfulness and being aware of your physical and mental state allows you to better handle the pressures that may arise during emergencies.

Acupressure is another alternative health practice that can be useful for preppers. This involves applying pressure to certain points on the body to relieve pain, improve circulation, and support organ health. For example, pressing between the thumb and index finger can help relieve headaches, while pressing certain points on the wrist can reduce nausea. Acupressure is a simple and effective practice that doesn't require any equipment, making it ideal for situations where resources are limited.

In terms of diet, natural remedies can be enhanced by including nutrient-dense foods that promote overall health. Eating a diet rich in fruits, vegetables, whole grains, and lean proteins provides essential vitamins and minerals that support all bodily functions. Foods high in fiber support digestion, while leafy greens provide iron and calcium. Omega-3 fatty acids, found in fish and flaxseeds, support brain health and reduce inflammation. Keeping a balanced diet is one of the best ways to ensure long-term health and wellness.

Fermented foods like yogurt, sauerkraut, and kimchi are also beneficial for gut health. They contain probiotics, which are healthy bacteria that support digestion and strengthen the immune system. By adding fermented foods to your diet, you help balance the gut microbiome, which is essential for overall health. If storing these foods isn't possible, probiotic supplements can also be beneficial for maintaining a healthy digestive system.

For skin health, natural oils and herbs can be used to keep skin clean and prevent infection. Aloe vera is excellent for soothing burns, cuts, and skin irritation. It has cooling properties that reduce inflammation and speed up healing. Calendula is another herb that can be used for skin health; it's anti-inflammatory and can be applied as a salve to treat minor wounds and rashes. Caring for skin health with these natural remedies is easy and can prevent complications that may arise from untreated skin issues.

Staying hydrated is one of the simplest yet most essential health practices. Water is necessary for every function in the body, from digestion to circulation. In emergencies, water sources may be limited, so it's crucial to have a water purification method and store clean water if possible. Herbal teas made from mint, chamomile, or lemon balm can also provide hydration while offering additional health benefits. Staying hydrated supports all other health practices and is a cornerstone of good health.

By understanding and incorporating natural remedies and alternative health practices, preppers can create a well-rounded approach to health and wellness. Herbs, essential oils, and holistic practices like acupressure and meditation are accessible and effective tools. They empower you to care for your body in times when conventional healthcare might not be an option. Building a natural health kit with key herbs, oils, and remedies provides peace of mind and equips you to handle various health challenges with confidence.

CHAPTER 9

Community Building and Networking

Why Community Networks Are Vital for Survival

Building a strong community network is essential for survival, especially in times of crisis. When people come together, they can pool resources, share skills, and offer emotional support, which can make all the difference during difficult times. In emergency situations, having a network of trusted people provides a safety net that can help individuals not only survive but also stay resilient and hopeful. A community can help with practical needs like food, water, and shelter, as well as provide companionship, encouragement, and a sense of belonging, all of which are critical for mental and emotional well-being.

One of the primary benefits of a community network is the sharing of resources. In a survival situation, resources like food, water, medical supplies, and tools may become limited or inaccessible. When people work together, they can distribute these resources more effectively. For example, if one person has a large stockpile of food but lacks water purification equipment, and another has an ample water supply but needs food, they can trade or share to ensure everyone's needs are met. This mutual exchange reduces individual burdens and increases the chances of survival for the entire group. A community can also collectively decide on rationing systems to make sure resources last as long as possible.

Skills sharing is another significant advantage of community building. Different people bring various skills and knowledge that can be invaluable in an emergency. Some might have medical training, while others are skilled in cooking, gardening, or mechanics. By combining these abilities, the group becomes much more capable and resourceful. For instance, a person skilled in first aid can handle medical needs, while another with building skills can help construct shelters or repair damaged equipment. This teamwork means that tasks can be done faster and more efficiently, providing a greater sense of security for everyone involved.

In addition to resources and skills, emotional support is a key reason why community networks are vital for survival. Facing a crisis alone can be isolating, frightening, and stressful. People often feel more capable of handling difficulties when they have others to lean on and talk to. Being able to share fears, offer encouragement, or simply spend time together can strengthen resilience and keep morale high. A network of supportive individuals can help people stay calm and clear-headed, which is essential for making wise decisions under pressure. Emotional connections reduce feelings of loneliness and helplessness, making it easier to stay motivated and hopeful.

Community networks also enhance safety and security. In emergencies, there is often a need for defense against threats, whether from natural disasters or human dangers. A group of people working together can establish patrols, keep watch, and create safety protocols. Individuals are less vulnerable when they are part of a group that can protect each other. Shared vigilance and planning make it harder for external threats to disrupt the community, providing a safer environment for all members. People can take turns resting while others keep watch, ensuring constant protection and enabling everyone to conserve energy.

Another advantage of community networks is the potential for learning and skill-building. When people with different backgrounds come together, they can teach each other essential survival skills, which makes the entire group stronger. For example, one person may know how to fish, while another understands how to identify edible plants. By teaching each other, they expand the group's collective knowledge, which can be lifesaving. Regular practice of skills like fire-making, shelter-building, and first aid can also prepare the group for unexpected situations. This shared knowledge builds confidence, as each person becomes more capable and prepared.

Beyond survival, community networks allow for the possibility of rebuilding or adapting to a new normal. After the immediate crisis has passed, a strong community can work together to rebuild, create new systems, or adapt to new living conditions. People can start growing food, creating sustainable water sources, and setting up a system for trading or bartering. Rebuilding as a group is much easier than doing it alone, as everyone can contribute according to their abilities and resources. A community network offers a path to recovery, stability, and even a better quality of life, helping individuals regain a sense of control and purpose.

In community networks, trust is essential. Trusting one another means that individuals feel safe sharing resources, relying on others for support, and working together toward shared goals. Building trust within a group takes time, open communication, and reliability. When people feel that they can depend on each other, they are more likely to make sacrifices for the benefit of the whole. Trust encourages collaboration and reduces conflicts, making the group more cohesive and resilient. Community members need to communicate openly, respect one another's contributions, and demonstrate accountability to maintain this trust.

Planning and organizing within a community network is crucial to its effectiveness. Roles and responsibilities should be defined, ensuring that each person knows their duties and can perform them when needed. Leaders can be chosen to guide the group, coordinate resources, and make decisions. However, it is also important for everyone to have a voice in planning to feel included and committed to the group's goals. Regular meetings, where people can discuss concerns and strategies, help maintain unity and keep everyone informed. Good organization maximizes efficiency, reduces misunderstandings, and enables the group to respond quickly to changing circumstances.

Community networks are also beneficial for information-sharing. In times of crisis, staying informed about current events, weather conditions, and other developments is essential. Members of a community can share updates, news, and observations that help everyone stay aware of potential dangers or opportunities. This collective knowledge allows the group to make better decisions based on the most recent and reliable information. Whether through radios, word-of-mouth, or other means, a well-connected community has an advantage in adapting to new challenges.

Community networks provide opportunities for children, elderly individuals, and others who may be more vulnerable. In a crisis, these individuals can receive the care and attention they need through the collective efforts of the group. Families can rely on each other to look after children, help with physical tasks, or provide extra support for those with specific needs. This support system ensures that everyone is taken care of and has a role to play, even if they cannot contribute as actively as others. By valuing and protecting each member, the community network fosters a sense of unity and shared purpose.

Community networks are crucial for preppers and survivalists because they bring together resources, skills, and emotional support that individuals would struggle to maintain alone. By pooling resources, sharing expertise, providing emotional resilience, enhancing security, and fostering learning, a well-connected group can navigate crises more effectively and emerge stronger. These networks build trust, promote effective organization, and ensure that even vulnerable members are supported. Building a community network isn't just about survival; it's about creating a resilient, supportive environment where people can work together, face challenges, and find hope, even in the toughest of times. A strong community is one of the most valuable assets for anyone preparing for the uncertainties of the future.

Forming Survival Groups and Mutual Aid Agreements

Forming survival groups and establishing mutual aid agreements can be essential for effective preparedness and survival in times of crisis. Working together with trusted individuals allows you to pool resources, share skills, and build a support system that is stronger and more resilient than what one person could achieve alone. By creating survival groups and building partnerships with others, you not only improve your own chances of enduring difficult situations but also contribute to a larger network of safety and support.

Survival groups can start by bringing together people with common goals and values. These are individuals who understand the importance of preparedness and are willing to contribute their time, resources, and skills. It's important to select group members carefully, considering factors like trustworthiness, reliability, and commitment to the group's goals. Friends, family members, neighbors, or even local community members who share similar outlooks on survival can make good group members. A shared understanding and open communication are essential to ensure everyone is on the same page and committed to working together.

Once a group is formed, it's helpful to hold regular meetings to discuss preparedness plans, roles, and responsibilities. This allows each member to understand their role in the group, creating a sense of accountability and dependability. Roles might include things like medical support, security, resource management, and communications. For instance, someone with a medical background could take responsibility for first aid and medical supplies, while another with experience in mechanics might handle tools and equipment. Assigning roles helps the group operate efficiently and makes sure that essential needs are covered.

Pooling resources is one of the biggest benefits of forming a survival group. By combining what each person can contribute, the group can build a stronger stockpile than any individual could on their own. This might include food, water, medical supplies, tools, and even things like fuel or vehicles. Having a shared resource pool means that everyone in the group has access to critical supplies during a crisis, reducing the chances of anyone going without basic necessities. It's also a good idea to keep an inventory of all the shared resources so that the group knows what is available and can plan accordingly.

One important aspect of forming a survival group is discussing and establishing rules and guidelines. A clear agreement on how resources will be shared, how decisions will be made, and how conflicts will be resolved can prevent misunderstandings and disputes. These guidelines create a sense of fairness and structure within the group, allowing everyone to feel secure and know what to expect. Rules can cover things like how often members should contribute supplies, how they will be distributed, and how group decisions will be handled, either by voting or consensus.

Mutual aid agreements with neighbors and friends are another effective way to extend your preparedness network. Mutual aid involves a commitment to assist each other in times of need, whether it's with physical resources, skills, or emotional support. You might arrange to share supplies like food, water, or medical equipment, or you might agree to assist each other in specific tasks, like security or evacuation. These agreements are especially helpful because they build a sense of community and allow you to work together with people who may live nearby, making it easier to coordinate efforts.

When establishing a mutual aid agreement, it's beneficial to meet with the other parties and openly discuss what each person or household can offer. For example, if you have experience in gardening and can produce extra food, you might offer to share that food with a neighbor who has medical training and can help in a health emergency. The goal is to create an arrangement where each party brings something valuable to the table, making the collective network stronger and more resilient.

A major benefit of collaborative prepping is that it provides a wider range of skills and knowledge. Different people bring unique expertise to the group, which increases the group's overall ability to handle different aspects of survival. For example, one person might be skilled in water purification, another in first aid, and someone else in mechanics. When you combine these skills, the group has the tools to tackle various challenges without having to rely on any single individual. This also allows each person to focus on their strengths and learn from others, making the group better prepared as a whole.

Communication is crucial when working with a survival group or within mutual aid agreements. Good communication helps prevent misunderstandings and ensures that everyone knows what's happening within the group. Regular check-ins, meetings, or even simple updates through text messages can keep everyone informed. It's also helpful to have a way to communicate during emergencies, such as walkie-talkies or radios, so that group members can stay in touch even if phone lines or the internet are down.

Security and safety are other important considerations in survival groups and mutual aid arrangements. When you have a trusted group, it becomes easier to organize a secure perimeter, take turns standing guard, or watch over each other's homes. Working as a group can provide additional security for everyone involved, as there is strength in numbers. The group can establish security protocols, such as rotating shifts or having a plan for signaling each other in case of danger. This kind of organized approach to safety helps everyone feel more secure and enables them to focus on other survival tasks.

Establishing a written plan or agreement can help solidify the commitment among group members. This document can outline each person's responsibilities, the resources they are contributing, and the expectations for behavior. It can also include contingency plans, like what to do if someone is unable to contribute or if a member needs to leave the group. While a formal document may not be necessary for every group, it can serve as a helpful reference that reduces misunderstandings and reinforces everyone's commitment.

Flexibility and adaptability are key traits for successful survival groups. Emergencies are often unpredictable, and a rigid plan may not work in every situation. Group members should be willing to adapt and make changes as needed, responding to new challenges with creativity and cooperation. Having an open-minded approach and being willing to listen to each other's ideas can lead to better solutions and help the group stay resilient in the face of unexpected situations.

Building alliances with neighbors and friends is particularly valuable in rural or isolated areas, where outside help may be slow to arrive. In these settings, mutual aid and survival groups can form the backbone of a community's emergency response. By building trust and cooperation with those around you, you create a local support system that is ready to assist during times of need. These alliances help people remain self-sufficient and ensure that everyone has a backup network when resources are scarce or professional help is unavailable.

Involving children, elderly members, and others who may need additional assistance is also crucial in survival groups. Everyone should feel they have a role to play, even if it's something small, like helping with food preparation or watching over the younger kids. Assigning age-appropriate tasks ensures that everyone is contributing to the group's efforts and helps build a sense of unity. It's essential to consider any special needs that group members might have and plan accordingly, so everyone can be taken care of and kept safe.

Forming survival groups and creating mutual aid agreements can greatly enhance your preparedness and chances of survival. These groups allow for resource pooling, skills sharing, and the emotional support needed to handle stressful situations. Establishing rules, planning for security, and encouraging open communication all contribute to a strong, resilient group. When people come together in these ways, they create a network of trust and support that is vital for survival in uncertain times. By working collaboratively, you and your group can build a foundation of strength and readiness, prepared to face whatever challenges may come.

Contributing to Local Resilience in Times of Crisis

Contributing to local resilience during a crisis is one of the most valuable ways preppers can support their communities. By sharing knowledge, resources, and skills, preppers not only help those around them but also strengthen the overall ability of their community to survive difficult times. This creates a ripple effect, where cooperation and preparedness multiply, and everyone benefits. In times of crisis, individuals who can lead, work together, and show compassion create a foundation of support that can make a critical difference.

Sharing knowledge is one of the simplest yet most impactful contributions a prepper can make to their community. Many people may lack essential survival skills, such as purifying water, growing food, or providing basic first aid. A prepper with experience in these areas can teach these skills to others, helping them become more self-reliant and less vulnerable in a crisis. For example, setting up workshops or classes on food preservation or home gardening allows community members to gain practical skills that support their long-term well-being. Preppers can also distribute handouts or share online guides with step-by-step instructions on various survival techniques. By educating others, preppers equip their neighbors with the tools needed to handle emergencies with greater confidence.

In addition to skills, sharing resources when possible also strengthens local resilience. During crises, certain resources such as clean water, food, and medical supplies become especially scarce. Preppers who have built up a reserve of these supplies may consider helping others by sharing or lending items as needed. For instance, if a prepper has access to a water purification system, they might offer purified water to those who need it or teach neighbors how to purify water themselves. Sharing doesn't mean giving away everything, but it does involve a willingness to help in a way that protects the entire community. When people know they can count on each other for support, everyone feels safer and more secure, which helps prevent panic.

Building strong relationships with neighbors before a crisis happens can also contribute to community resilience. Preppers can get to know their neighbors, learn about their needs and strengths, and build a sense of trust. These relationships form the foundation of effective cooperation during difficult times. For example, a community where people already know each other well is more likely to work together effectively to share resources, protect each other's homes, and provide mutual aid. By actively connecting with their community, preppers foster a spirit of togetherness that becomes incredibly valuable when challenges arise.

Leadership plays a key role in building community resilience. Preppers can provide calm and knowledgeable guidance, helping others stay organized and focused during a crisis. Effective leaders listen to concerns, encourage cooperation, and make sure people feel included in decision-making processes. They create a sense of order and direction, which reduces fear and confusion. For example, a prepper who has experience in crisis management can help organize community meetings to discuss safety, distribute resources fairly, or set up a plan for neighborhood watch. Good leaders inspire confidence and trust, allowing people to pull together as a team and manage challenges with a positive attitude.

Cooperation within the community is essential during emergencies. When people work together, they can accomplish much more than any individual could on their own. Preppers who promote cooperation can help organize teams for specific tasks, such as security patrols, food distribution, or cleanup efforts. In addition, preppers can foster an environment where everyone's skills and contributions are valued. This might include organizing groups to help with gardening, carpentry, or cooking, based on each person's strengths. By encouraging teamwork, preppers create an atmosphere where everyone contributes to the community's well-being, which increases morale and resilience.

In times of crisis, charity and kindness become even more important. While self-preservation is essential, extending help to those who are struggling can strengthen bonds and uplift the entire community. For preppers, charity might mean helping elderly neighbors who need extra support, assisting families with young children, or providing comfort to those who are scared or anxious. These acts of kindness do not have to be grand; even small gestures can make a significant difference. For instance, sharing extra food, offering a comforting conversation, or providing blankets and clothing to those in need can ease others' suffering and foster a sense of hope. In challenging times, compassion goes a long way in building a supportive community.

Preppers who are skilled in alternative forms of communication, such as radio, can also offer an essential service to their community by helping maintain contact with the outside world. When normal communication networks fail, radio operators can relay news, weather updates, and important announcements. By setting up a central communication point, preppers can ensure that their community stays informed, reducing fear and helping people make better decisions based on reliable information.

Another way preppers can contribute is by organizing mutual aid agreements with other communities. If one neighborhood has access to fresh water but lacks medical supplies, while another has medicine but limited food, preppers can arrange exchanges that benefit both sides. This type of cooperation allows communities to share resources they have in abundance with those who lack them, creating a mutually beneficial relationship. Preppers who encourage these types of alliances help ensure that resources are distributed more evenly, which increases everyone's chances of surviving difficult times.

Maintaining mental health is another crucial aspect of resilience that preppers can support in their communities. During crises, stress, anxiety, and fear can take a toll on people's mental well-being.

Preppers who have learned techniques for managing stress, such as breathing exercises, meditation, or mindfulness, can share these practices with others. Additionally, simply being a calm and positive presence can help others feel more secure. Preppers who offer emotional support, either through listening or offering words of encouragement, play a vital role in helping their community stay mentally strong.

Preppers can also play a role in teaching self-sufficiency skills that go beyond emergency preparedness. Skills such as cooking from scratch, building repairs, and basic agriculture are useful for long-term resilience, not only during a crisis. Offering classes, demonstrations, or even one-on-one guidance on these skills helps empower others to be more self-reliant. When more people in a community can cook, repair, and grow their own food, the community as a whole becomes more resilient and less dependent on outside help.

In addition, preppers who are knowledgeable about health and hygiene practices can contribute to preventing the spread of illness. During crises, simple hygiene practices like regular hand-washing, safe food storage, and waste disposal become even more critical to maintaining health. Preppers can share knowledge on these practices and distribute basic hygiene supplies, such as soap and disinfectant, if they have extras. Preventing illness helps reduce the strain on community resources and keeps people healthy, making it easier to handle other aspects of the crisis.

Fostering hope and resilience is perhaps one of the most powerful contributions preppers can make. By setting an example of preparedness, calm, and confidence, they inspire others to adopt a proactive approach to challenges. When people see that they have the ability to prepare and respond effectively, they feel more empowered and less vulnerable. Preppers who encourage this mindset help create a community where people face difficulties with courage and resilience.

Preppers can play a transformative role in building local resilience by sharing knowledge, resources, and skills with their community. Through leadership, cooperation, and compassion, they help create a network of support that benefits everyone. In times of crisis, these contributions make the community stronger, safer, and more united. Working together, communities can face adversity with the confidence that they have the skills, resources, and support needed to survive and even thrive.

CHAPTER 10

Long-Term Sustainability

Defining Long-Term Sustainability in the Prepper Context

Long-term sustainability is essential for anyone preparing for emergencies, as it focuses on creating a lifestyle that can endure over time, even in difficult conditions. For preppers, long-term sustainability means adopting practices and strategies that allow for continued survival without relying heavily on outside resources. It involves developing ways to meet essential needs; such as food, water, shelter, and energy that do not deplete resources too quickly or harm the environment, making them renewable and self-sustaining. By building self-sufficiency, preppers become more resilient to disruptions, from temporary crises to extended emergencies, while reducing vulnerability to shortages or supply chain breakdowns.

A key aspect of long-term sustainability is food security. Growing one's food, whether through gardening, raising animals, or both, provides a stable source of nourishment that does not depend on grocery stores or outside suppliers. Small-scale farming, if done properly, allows preppers to produce crops year-round, storing food through preservation techniques like canning or drying for times when fresh produce may not be available. A sustainable garden not only provides food but also saves money and energy that would otherwise be spent on obtaining food from faraway sources. It creates a closed-loop system where nutrients are recycled, plants are rotated to maintain soil health, and natural methods are used to minimize waste.

Water is another essential component of long-term sustainability. In a self-sustaining setup, having a reliable water source and a way to purify it is crucial. Many preppers create rainwater collection systems, capturing water that can be filtered and used for drinking, gardening, and hygiene. This water supply can be managed to ensure it lasts even during dry periods. Additionally, maintaining a well or other freshwater source close to home provides independence from municipal water systems, which could be compromised in a crisis. Proper water management is not just about having enough water; it's about using it wisely and efficiently to meet daily needs without exhausting the supply.

Energy sustainability is also critical. Preppers who rely solely on traditional electricity grids may find themselves in a challenging situation if those grids fail. Sustainable energy sources, like solar panels, wind turbines, and even small-scale hydropower setups, allow for reliable, renewable power that isn't vulnerable to outages. Solar energy, for example, provides an ongoing power supply as long as there is sunlight, enabling preppers to cook, light their homes, and power essential devices without worrying about access to gas or electricity. Although setting up alternative energy sources may require an initial investment, they prove invaluable over time by providing consistent power and reducing reliance on external suppliers.

Reducing waste is another core part of long-term sustainability. A sustainable prepper lifestyle minimizes waste by reusing, repurposing, and recycling as much as possible. Instead of throwing away items that may still have uses, preppers can find creative ways to repurpose materials. For example, glass jars can store food, plastic containers can be used for gardening, and composting can turn food scraps into valuable soil amendments. By adopting a mindset of waste reduction, preppers not only create less trash but also conserve resources, making what they have last longer and reducing the need to rely on outside supplies.

Sustainable practices also involve using renewable resources instead of finite ones. Preppers can focus on building systems that rely on naturally replenished materials, like using wood for heat from sustainably managed forests rather than relying on fossil fuels. Sustainable hunting, fishing, and foraging allow preppers to source food without putting excessive strain on local ecosystems, ensuring these resources are available in the future. Using renewable resources means thinking about the long-term impact of actions and making choices that do not deplete the environment, which is vital for those aiming to sustain their lifestyle over an extended period.

Preparedness also includes developing practical skills that support self-sufficiency, from cooking and preserving food to making clothing and repairing tools. Knowledge of skills like carpentry, mechanics, and first aid can make a significant difference in a prepper's ability to remain self-reliant. Rather than depending on outside help, people with these skills can fix their belongings, build necessary structures, and care for their own health needs. These abilities empower preppers to be resilient and adaptable, helping them overcome challenges that would otherwise force them to seek outside assistance.

Community cooperation is an often-overlooked but essential aspect of sustainability. When preppers work together with their neighbors or nearby communities, they can share resources, skills, and labor, making long-term survival more manageable for everyone. By forming alliances, groups can rotate tasks, share expertise, and create a support network that increases the sustainability of their way of life. A prepper who is skilled in medicine, for example, could provide health care to others in exchange for goods or services they lack. This shared approach to sustainability makes it possible for everyone in the group to thrive while reducing the stress of having to do everything alone.

Mental and emotional well-being is also a part of sustainable preparedness. Crises, especially prolonged ones, can take a toll on mental health, and it's important to have coping strategies that help maintain morale and resilience. Sustainable preppers find ways to nurture a positive mindset, whether through meditation, journaling, or community support. In a long-term survival scenario, keeping spirits high and maintaining hope play critical roles in sustaining energy and motivation. Mental preparedness, in this sense, means developing a resilient mindset that can handle stress, adapt to change, and stay focused on survival goals, which are essential traits for facing prolonged challenges.

Embracing sustainability ultimately means creating a balanced approach to preparedness. It's about preparing not only for immediate needs but for ongoing self-sufficiency that conserves resources, protects the environment, and ensures continuity. For example, permaculture is a sustainable gardening practice that mimics natural ecosystems, ensuring food production in a way that regenerates the soil and preserves biodiversity. Implementing permaculture principles in food production can yield long-lasting benefits, providing food while enriching the land rather than depleting it. By cultivating a balanced approach that respects nature, preppers contribute to the health of the land and resources they depend on.

Sustainable practices not only enhance resilience but also reduce dependence on external systems, providing a stable, reliable way of life that isn't at risk from interruptions or scarcity. When preppers cultivate their own food, harness renewable energy, and build a lifestyle that reuses and recycles resources, they gain control over their survival. This independence allows them to withstand challenges that others may find overwhelming, as they are not as reliant on external resources. Over time, this level of self-sufficiency brings security and peace of mind, as sustainable preppers know they can endure adversity without depending on factors outside their control.

Incorporating sustainability into prepping is not just about surviving; it's about thriving. By focusing on renewable resources, developing self-sufficiency skills, and building strong community networks, preppers can create a lifestyle that promotes long-term stability. Sustainable practices ensure that resources will continue to be available, making it possible to meet needs without exhausting supplies. This resilience is a powerful asset, as it enables preppers to approach any challenge with the confidence that they have built a foundation strong enough to endure.

Long-term sustainability in the prepper context is about creating a life that is as self-reliant and resilient as possible, using practices that respect resources and prioritize renewal. Sustainable practices enable preppers to live in a way that minimizes reliance on external systems and maximizes self-sufficiency, making them well-prepared for any situation. By adopting these practices, preppers not only enhance their chances of survival but contribute to a more balanced, eco-friendly approach that benefits them and their communities. Sustainability, at its core, is about building a secure future, one that's adaptable, enduring, and resourceful.

Off-Grid Energy and Sustainable Living Solutions

Off-grid energy options and sustainable living practices are important tools for creating a self-reliant lifestyle. Living "off-grid" means being able to meet essential needs like electricity, water, and waste management without depending on external systems. This can be useful in times of crisis, but it also allows people to live more eco-friendly lives, with less impact on the environment. Solar, wind, and hydro power are three of the most popular ways to generate energy off the grid, each with its unique benefits. Together with sustainable practices like water harvesting, waste management, and green building, these systems provide a foundation for a life that is independent and aligned with nature.

Solar power is one of the most accessible forms of off-grid energy, as it relies on sunlight to generate electricity. Solar panels, which are the devices that capture sunlight, convert the sun's energy into electricity that can power lights, appliances, and other devices. One of the best things about solar power is its simplicity: once the panels are installed, they provide a steady supply of energy without ongoing fuel costs or pollution. Solar panels work best in sunny areas, but even in cloudy or colder climates, they can still produce electricity. Solar energy can also be stored in batteries, allowing people to use it even at night or during cloudy days. While solar systems may require a higher initial investment, they are cost-effective over time, reducing or even eliminating electricity bills.

Wind power is another valuable option, especially in areas with consistent, strong winds. Small wind turbines can be installed on properties to generate electricity by capturing the energy of moving air. Like solar, wind power is renewable and doesn't pollute, and it can also complement solar energy well: while solar panels produce less energy during cloudy or rainy days, wind turbines may generate more power during these times. Wind turbines work by using blades that spin in the wind to drive a generator, producing electricity. For homes or small communities, this can be an efficient way to stay powered. However, wind energy depends on the location, as areas with little wind won't produce enough power to make it worthwhile. Properly setting up and maintaining a wind turbine does take skill and sometimes assistance, but for those in windy regions, it's a reliable and sustainable choice.

Hydro power, which uses the energy of flowing water, is another effective off-grid energy solution. Hydro systems are typically installed near rivers or streams where water flows steadily. When water flows through a small turbine, it spins the turbine's blades, generating electricity. This type of system is especially beneficial because water flows constantly, providing a more continuous source of energy compared to solar and wind. Hydro systems are efficient and can power entire homes or communities if there is enough flowing water available. However, they are more limited by location since a water source is required, and setting up a hydro system can involve complex installation. But for those near a reliable stream or river, hydro power is a powerful and consistent energy solution that works even when the sun isn't shining or the wind isn't blowing.

Alongside energy generation, sustainable water harvesting is crucial for off-grid living. One common method is rainwater harvesting, where rainwater is collected from rooftops or other surfaces and stored in tanks for future use. This collected water can be filtered and used for drinking, cooking, cleaning, or watering plants. Rainwater harvesting is a simple but effective way to have a renewable water source, especially in areas with regular rainfall. Proper filtration is essential for making rainwater safe to drink, as it may contain contaminants from the roof or air. Storing water in clean, covered containers also helps prevent contamination. For those in areas with little rain, other methods like digging a well or installing a hand pump can provide alternative sources of water, though it's important to ensure that the water source is safe and regularly tested.

Waste management is another vital part of sustainable, off-grid living. Proper waste disposal keeps the environment clean and reduces health risks. Composting is a popular way to manage food scraps and organic waste, turning it into a natural fertilizer that can be used in gardens. This not only reduces landfill waste but also enriches the soil with nutrients. Composting systems can be as simple as a bin in the backyard where food scraps and yard waste break down over time. Toilets designed for off-grid use, like composting or dry toilets, handle human waste by turning it into compost or separating liquids from solids. These options are safer for the environment, as they don't require water to flush, saving resources and preventing pollution.

Green building techniques focus on designing and constructing homes that are energy-efficient, environmentally friendly, and comfortable. For example, using natural materials like stone, clay, or bamboo reduces reliance on industrially produced building materials, which often use a lot of energy to manufacture. Straw bale houses are one example of green building, where straw bales are used for insulation, making homes naturally warm in winter and cool in summer. Green roofs, which involve growing plants on rooftops, also provide insulation and reduce heating and cooling needs, while also helping to manage rainwater. Homes can be oriented to maximize sunlight for passive heating, where large windows on south-facing walls let in sunlight, warming the home without additional heating. These practices reduce energy needs and create a comfortable living environment that works with nature.

Another sustainable building approach is to design homes that work well with renewable energy systems. Homes can be wired to be energy-efficient by using energy-saving appliances, LED lighting, and efficient heating and cooling systems. This reduces the demand on solar panels, wind turbines, or hydro systems, making it easier to meet energy needs with renewable sources. Designing homes to be smaller and more efficient, without wasted space, further reduces energy consumption, making off-grid living more sustainable and comfortable.

Sustainable off-grid living is also about cultivating habits that reduce overall consumption. Simple changes, like reducing unnecessary lighting, using energy-efficient devices, and making use of natural sunlight whenever possible, contribute to a more sustainable lifestyle. Planning meals to minimize waste, preserving food through canning or drying, and reusing containers and packaging materials are small but impactful ways to live sustainably. Reducing dependence on single-use items, conserving water by fixing leaks, and installing low-flow fixtures all help conserve valuable resources, making off-grid living easier to manage over time.

By combining these off-grid energy solutions and sustainable practices, people can create a life that is self-sufficient and resilient. Solar, wind, and hydro power provide renewable energy options that work in harmony with nature, while water harvesting and waste management ensure essential resources are handled responsibly. Green building techniques and mindful consumption create homes that are efficient and comfortable. Off-grid and sustainable living requires effort and planning, but by adopting these practices, people can live more independently and in closer alignment with the natural world. This lifestyle not only reduces environmental impact but also provides a secure foundation that is less reliant on outside resources, making it a valuable choice for anyone seeking self-sufficiency and resilience.

Permaculture and Homesteading for Self-Sufficiency

Permaculture and homesteading are valuable practices that can support long-term self-sufficiency by integrating sustainable methods into everyday life. Both practices aim to create a balanced, natural environment that can continuously support human needs without exhausting resources. Permaculture is a system of agriculture that works with nature, promoting biodiversity, healthy soil, and renewable energy. Homesteading, on the other hand, focuses on living off the land, often through growing food, raising animals, and reducing reliance on store-bought goods. By combining these approaches, people can create a sustainable living environment that supports itself and reduces dependence on outside resources.

Permaculture focuses on designing a living space that mimics the natural ecosystem, using plants and animals in a way that benefits the environment. It involves thoughtful planning to ensure each part of the ecosystem supports others. For example, a permaculture garden includes different types of plants that help each other grow. Trees might provide shade for shade-loving plants, while vines climb up the trees, making efficient use of space. Groundcover plants reduce soil erosion, retain moisture, and prevent weeds from taking over. This layering of plants, known as "stacking," ensures that every inch of the garden is productive, similar to how plants naturally grow in the wild.

Permaculture gardens also use compost and organic materials to improve soil quality. Healthy soil is essential for growing nutritious food, and composting provides a natural fertilizer. By recycling kitchen scraps and yard waste into compost, nutrients are returned to the soil, supporting plants without needing chemical fertilizers. Soil health can also be improved with crop rotation, where different crops are planted in various parts of the garden each year. This practice prevents the depletion of specific nutrients and helps reduce pests and diseases that might thrive if the same plants were grown in the same spot repeatedly. Additionally, using mulch made of straw, leaves, or wood chips helps retain moisture and keeps the soil cool, reducing the need for watering.

Growing food in a permaculture garden is central to self-sufficiency. People often begin with easy-to-grow vegetables, fruits, and herbs, choosing plants that thrive in their climate and soil type. Perennial plants, like asparagus, rhubarb, and certain herbs, are especially useful because they grow back year after year without replanting. Fruit trees and berry bushes also provide ongoing harvests. By planning for a mix of crops that mature at different times, a permaculture garden can provide fresh food year-round. This practice, called succession planting, ensures a steady supply of produce throughout the seasons and reduces the need for long-term storage.

Homesteading adds another dimension to self-sufficiency by incorporating animals into the ecosystem. Animals like chickens, goats, rabbits, and bees contribute food, provide fertilizer, and support the overall health of the land. Chickens, for example, lay eggs, eat pests, and produce manure that can be composted to enrich the soil. Goats can supply milk, which can be used to make cheese, butter, and yogurt, and they help clear weeds. Bees are valuable for pollinating plants, leading to better yields of fruits and vegetables. Raising animals on a homestead requires proper care, shelter, and knowledge, but the benefits they bring to a sustainable environment make them worthwhile.

Permaculture and homesteading also emphasize water conservation and efficient water use. Collecting rainwater in barrels or cisterns provides a renewable water source for gardens and animals. Drip irrigation systems, which deliver water directly to the roots of plants, reduce water waste and keep plants healthier. Graywater systems, which reuse water from sinks, showers, and washing machines, can also be implemented to irrigate plants. By managing water carefully, a homestead can stay resilient even in dry periods, and plants and animals continue to thrive without relying on city water.

Creating a sustainable living environment goes beyond just producing food and conserving water; it also involves managing waste responsibly. Permaculture encourages the use of waste as a resource, recycling materials back into the ecosystem. Composting food scraps, animal waste, and yard debris turns waste into rich soil. Other waste, like paper, wood, or natural fibers, can be reused in various ways, such as making mulch, insulation, or animal bedding. Even small practices, like reusing containers for planting or repairing tools, reduce waste and make homesteading more self-sustaining.

Natural building techniques are another part of creating a sustainable living space. Homes can be constructed using locally sourced and renewable materials like straw, mud, wood, and stone. These materials are often more environmentally friendly and less costly than traditional construction. Straw bale walls, for example, provide excellent insulation, keeping homes warm in winter and cool in summer. Earth-based construction, like adobe or cob, also has natural insulating properties and blends well with the landscape. These building techniques not only save money and energy but also align with permaculture principles, creating harmony between human structures and nature.

Permaculture and homesteading both place importance on renewable energy. Solar panels, wind turbines, and small hydroelectric systems are popular choices for powering off-grid homes. By generating power on-site, a homestead reduces its dependence on external sources and lowers its carbon footprint. Energy conservation is also key; using energy-efficient appliances, LED lighting, and passive heating and cooling strategies like shaded windows or ventilation reduces the amount of energy needed. Sustainable energy choices further enhance self-sufficiency and make a homestead more resilient to disruptions in external power supplies.

The skills learned through permaculture and homesteading foster independence and adaptability. Knowing how to grow food, care for animals, conserve water, manage waste, and use renewable energy creates a foundation for resilience. These practices can be adjusted to meet specific needs, making them accessible even in small spaces. Community support is also an important part of these lifestyles, as people often share knowledge, trade goods, or help each other with tasks. By connecting with others who are interested in sustainable living, homesteaders and permaculture practitioners can learn from each other, creating a support network that extends their self-sufficiency.

Permaculture and homesteading offer more than just survival skills; they provide a way to live in harmony with nature and reduce environmental impact. These practices teach respect for natural resources, showing how each part of the ecosystem has a role to play. By applying permaculture design principles and homesteading skills, preppers can create a sustainable living environment that provides food, water, energy, and shelter while preserving the land for future generations. In this way, permaculture and homesteading are not only about surviving but also about building a fulfilling life that contributes to a healthier planet.

Through these practices, preppers can achieve a sustainable, independent lifestyle that aligns with nature's cycles. Growing food, raising animals, and building sustainably allows them to be less dependent on external systems, enhancing resilience and reducing vulnerability. With permaculture and homesteading, self-sufficiency becomes a practical reality, creating a lifestyle that values both personal well-being and the health of the environment.

CONCLUSION

Preparedness is a journey, a commitment to securing a safe, resilient, and sustainable future. Throughout this book, we have explored the tools, knowledge, and mindsets necessary for becoming prepared for life's unexpected turns. Each chapter has been filled with principles and strategies that can empower individuals and families to weather difficult times, maintain health, and establish a level of independence that is increasingly important in today's world. This is not just about stockpiling goods, but about learning lifelong skills that enhance self-reliance and provide security, even in the face of disruption.

Preparedness begins with understanding why it matters. Being prepared means having thought through potential emergencies, from natural disasters to economic challenges, and having plans in place to meet basic needs like food, water, shelter, and safety. We've discussed how important it is to have a personalized plan, one that reflects your location, family structure, and resources. By identifying vulnerabilities in advance, you are already taking steps toward securing your future.

Building self-sufficiency is a fundamental part of preparedness, reducing reliance on outside sources and ensuring you can provide for yourself and your family. By learning practical skills like food storage, gardening, animal husbandry, and preserving resources, self-sufficiency becomes achievable. Food security, in particular, plays a central role; growing your own food or having a solid food storage plan reduces dependency on grocery stores. Knowing how to safely store and rotate supplies ensures they remain usable and nutritious. This also provides peace of mind, knowing that you can meet basic nutritional needs even if external sources are unavailable.

Water, too, is crucial to survival and requires careful planning. We explored ways to source, filter, and conserve water, whether through rainwater harvesting or filtration systems. Having a reliable supply of clean water is one of the most critical aspects of preparedness, and understanding various techniques for sourcing and purifying water ensures that your family can stay hydrated and healthy, even when typical sources are interrupted.

Energy and warmth are additional key areas. With off-grid energy options like solar and wind power, individuals can reduce dependence on public utilities and develop a sustainable energy source that works in most climates. We discussed various options for heating, cooling, and powering a home, all with an eye toward sustainability and reliability. This ensures not only comfort but also the functionality of necessary devices, even in the absence of public utilities. Efficient use of energy also makes a prepared household more resilient and less vulnerable to changes in fuel or electricity availability.

We also looked into the importance of health and wellness in long-term survival. Maintaining physical health through balanced nutrition, regular exercise, and proper hygiene is vital for strength and resilience. Emergency situations are stressful, and caring for your mental well-being through stress-management techniques, mindfulness, and maintaining connections with others makes a difference. Knowledge of natural remedies and alternative health practices empowers you to handle minor ailments when professional care might not be readily accessible. Prioritizing both physical and mental health helps ensure that you have the endurance and focus needed to handle the challenges of a crisis.

Financial preparedness is another significant part of long-term planning. Securing finances through smart savings, budgeting, and diversifying assets protects against economic downturns or personal financial crises. Having cash on hand, reducing debt, and learning barter skills for times when money might lose its purchasing power allows for flexibility and adaptability. Financial resilience goes beyond accumulating wealth; it's about managing resources wisely, minimizing waste, and investing in skills, supplies, and tools that add value over time.

Community and connection were also emphasized. No one is truly alone in an emergency; strong community bonds provide emotional support, shared resources, and collective problem-solving. Forming networks and mutual aid agreements means that resources and skills are pooled, ensuring that each person has access to what they need and contributing to the group's overall resilience. Whether it's family, friends, or neighbors, these relationships reinforce the idea that preparedness is often most effective when it's done together.

For those who wish to live a truly sustainable lifestyle, permaculture and homesteading offer a long-term solution to building a self-sufficient environment. By creating a system that naturally supports itself—through practices like gardening, raising animals, and recycling resources—a homestead can provide food, shelter, and energy sustainably. These methods, although more complex to establish, create a foundation for lasting independence and harmony with nature, ensuring that human needs are met without depleting the environment.

All of these aspects—preparedness, self-sufficiency, health, financial security, community, and sustainability—work together to form a well-rounded survival strategy. Together, they create a lifestyle that's not only resilient but fulfilling. This journey is about more than preparing for the worst; it's about building a life that's rich in skills, supportive relationships, and meaningful practices. It's a lifestyle that honors natural cycles, values human connection, and respects the land we depend on.

Taking action now is key. Begin by setting small, achievable goals, such as learning a new skill, storing a month's worth of food, or organizing a preparedness plan. Gradually build from there, gaining confidence and knowledge with each step. Even small actions make a difference. Remember that preparedness is a continuous process; it grows as you do, with each skill you learn, each resource you save, and each plan you make.

Preparedness also involves ongoing learning and adaptation. As your life changes or new challenges arise, revisit your plans, update your supplies, and refine your skills. Flexibility and adaptability are just as important as having supplies on hand. Keep in mind that the goal isn't perfection but progress. Each step you take strengthens your ability to handle whatever life brings your way.

Embracing preparedness empowers you to live with greater freedom and peace of mind. Knowing you're prepared allows you to focus on the present while feeling ready for the future. This readiness isn't just about having resources; it's about creating a balanced, resilient lifestyle that can sustain itself through difficulties. Ultimately, this journey prepares not only your home but also your mindset, equipping you with the confidence and resilience to thrive in a changing world.

Preparedness is both a choice and a commitment. By deciding to live with intention, forethought, and resourcefulness, you are creating a foundation for security, independence, and lasting well-being. Preparedness is a gift to yourself and to those around you, a proactive step toward a stable and empowered life. It is your path toward self-sufficiency, resilience, and a future where you can face challenges with courage and clarity.